Trauma-Informed Psychotherapy for BIPOC Communities

Grounded in trauma-informed approaches, intersectionality theory, and critical race theory, *Trauma-Informed Psychotherapy for BIPOC Communities: Decolonizing Mental Health* embodies psychotherapeutic practices via anti-racist, anti-oppressive, and culturally responsive paradigms.

Complete with practical case studies, psychoeducational frameworks, and the author's own inclusion and healing therapy (IHT) model, content from this book inspires practitioners to update their therapeutic competencies to effectively support BIPOC clients.

This book is an essential read for current and future intersectional psychologists, psychotherapists, social workers, counsellors, lawyers, educators, and healthcare professionals who actively work with BIPOC communities.

Pavna K. Sodhi, EdD (she/her), is a registered psychotherapist, author, and adjunct professor residing in Ontario, Canada. Dr. Sodhi's research spans over 25 years with specialization in immigrant and BIPOC mental health, multicultural counselling, and trauma-informed care. She credits her Punjabi-Sikh upbringing and lived experience for her continued interest in these timely topics. As a productive ally, she takes pride in decentring systemic racism, breaking barriers, and encouraging others to be culturally responsive.

"Dr. Sodhi effectively elucidates the impact on BIPOC of colonization, racism, and other dominating ideologies, presenting complex concepts in accessible ways, alongside practical strategies, and models for embracing a trauma-informed, anti-racist, anti-oppressive, culturally responsive approach to psychotherapy. Through her intentionally decolonizing language and unapologetic intent to abolish racism towards BIPOC communities, she both disrupts and decentres dominating eurocentric, colonial, and white supremacist approaches to health and healing. Readers will love the practical tips for enacting change in existing systems of oppression and for deepening awareness of the implications of their own embeddedness within these systems."

Sandra Collins, *PhD, RPsych, Researcher, Author, Consultant, and Curriculum Designer on Culturally Responsive and Socially Just Counselling, Victoria, British Columbia, Canada*

"An incredible book by Dr. Sodhi that brings together psychology, physiology, trauma and social justice in an engaging manner! Content is presented in a clear, applicable manner for clinicians in training, or seasoned clinicians looking to expand their therapeutic knowledge of diverse populations. Undoubtedly, this book is of significant importance in its contribution to the research literature given the inclusivity of content, BIPOC representation, and has wonderful potential to empower those who wish to help clients break systemic barriers."

Nita Tewari, *PhD, Founder and Licensed Psychologist at SITARA Psychology Center, Newport Beach, California, United States of America*

"Dr. Sodhi calls for a shift to decolonize professional practice beyond tokenistic aspiration. Her book offers a crucial nuancing of racial trauma and skillful application of her *Inclusion and Healing Therapy* Framework, convincing us that healing the pain of oppression cannot happen without personalized cultural attention. Irrefutably, professionals can no longer put off decolonizing their practice, and this book rightly encourages creating and holding that space as productive allies in anti-racism."

Cristelle Audet, *PhD, Registered Psychotherapist, Associate Professor, Co-editor of* Social Justice and Counselling: Discourse in Practice, *University of Ottawa, Ontario, Canada*

"A compelling and much-needed book for our times, when access to mental health resources for a growing and diverse population is needed more than ever, *Trauma-Informed Psychotherapy for BIPOC Communities: Decolonizing Mental Health* provides crucial insights on the effects of various forms of trauma and racism and how particular considerations in the healing process must be regarded for the well-being of our clients and our communities. Dr. Sodhi provides a comprehensive, yet concise background with clinical insights from her own healing journey and those of the numerous BIPOC clients she has served."

David Glickman, *MEd, Registered Psychotherapist, Algonquin College, Ottawa, Ontario, Canada*

Trauma-Informed Psychotherapy for BIPOC Communities

Decolonizing Mental Health

Pavna K. Sodhi, EdD

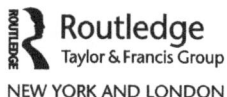
Routledge
Taylor & Francis Group

NEW YORK AND LONDON

Designed cover image: kastanka © Getty Images

First published 2024
by Routledge
605 Third Avenue, New York, NY 10158

and by Routledge
4 Park Square, Milton Park, Abingdon, Oxon, OX14 4RN

Routledge is an imprint of the Taylor & Francis Group, an informa business

© 2024 Pavna K. Sodhi

Library of Congress Cataloging-in-Publication Data
Names: Sodhi, Pavna K., author.
Title: Trauma-informed psychotherapy for BIPOC communities : decolonizing mental health / Pavna K. Sodhi.
Description: New York, NY : Routledge, 2024. | Includes bibliographical references and index.
Identifiers: LCCN 2023054798 (print) | LCCN 2023054799 (ebook) | ISBN 9781032106892 (hbk) | ISBN 9781032106854 (pbk) | ISBN 9781003216568 (ebk)
Subjects: LCSH: Psychotherapy. | Mental health.
Classification: LCC RC480 .S625 2024 (print) | LCC RC480 (ebook) | DDC 616.89/14—dc23/eng/20240117
LC record available at https://lccn.loc.gov/2023054798
LC ebook record available at https://lccn.loc.gov/2023054799

ISBN: 978-1-032-10689-2 (hbk)
ISBN: 978-1-032-10685-4 (pbk)
ISBN: 978-1-003-21656-8 (ebk)

DOI: 10.4324/9781003216568

Typeset in Sabon
by Apex CoVantage, LLC

To my maternal and paternal grandparents, who have taught me the value of cultural preservation and inner resilience.

To all BIPOC who have suffered and healed from systemic oppression and trauma.

Thank you for being cycle breakers.

This book is dedicated to you.

Contents

Illustrations

Figures

Tables

Credit List

Pavna K. Sodhi is appreciative for the permission to reprint the following texts and images:

Excerpt(s) from the poem "a hero" by Yung Pueblo first appeared in the poetry collection *Inward* copyright © 2018 by Diego Perez Lacera, published by Andrews McMeel Publishing.

The cycle of socialization by Bobbie Harro, from *Reading from Diversity and Social Justice* (edited by M. Adams, W. Blumenfeld, R. Castaneda, H. Hackman, M. Peters. & X. Zuniga), copyright © 2000, published by Taylor and Francis Group LLC (Books) US. Reproduced with permission of The Licensor through PLSclear.

Excerpt(s) from the introduction for emerging trends in multicultural psychotherapy by Pavna K. Sodhi. Used with permission of Taylor & Francis Group LLC – Books, from *Exploring Immigrant and Sexual Minority Mental Health: Reconsidering Multiculturalism*, Pavna K. Sodhi, © 2017, permission conveyed through Copyright Clearance Center, Inc.

The cycle of liberation by Bobbie Harro, from *Reading from Diversity and Social Justice* (edited by M. Adams, W. Blumenfeld, R. Castaneda, H. Hackman, M. Peters. & X. Zuniga), copyright © 2000, published by Taylor and Francis Group LLC (Books) US. Reproduced with permission of The Licensor through PLSclear.

Preface

A hero
is one who heals
their own wounds
and then shows others
how to do the same.

– Yung Pueblo
(*Inward*, 2018, p. 74)

Over a year ago, Katy Reinhardt introduced me to this resounding poem. I immediately felt it was the mantra of my book. During the authoring of my first book, without being able to name it, I experienced varying forms of trauma caused by marital discord, emotional abuse, and serious health issues (which I expand upon in my trauma narrative). What appeared to be my father's trauma response of immersing himself in his research eventually became mine. Academic and professional validation kept me afloat and in control of at least the career aspect of my life. To this day, conducting research and creative writing continue to be coping strategies or *glimmers* when I feel overwhelmed or activated.

While curating manuscript content, I seized the opportunity to "rewrite my narrative" (as I often suggest to clients) by enjoying the writing process without the same external stresses that transpired while prepared my first book. During this time, I asked myself: "Who would I be without my trauma?" In fact, my lived experience shaped the person I am today. It afforded me the platform to share my deep reflections regarding culturally responsive trauma-informed practices and strategies I have created for my BIPOC client caseload.

I understand and appreciate the complexities associated with trauma in BIPOC communities. As a collective, BIPOC may normalize or transmit trauma to future generations; however, we are in an era where these intergenerational cycles can be broken and smashed to release inner resilience, healing, and stamina. Healing from trauma requires first processing the unresolved traumatic events or experiences and then letting go of suffering, anger, and resentment; in short, sitting with one's emotions and renarrating one's story are inherently therapeutic. I hope this book inspires you, the reader, to reflect upon your trauma narrative, contemplate methods of individual and collective healing practices, and demonstrate to others how to heal from trauma.

Reference

Pueblo, Y. (2018) *Inward*. Andrews McMeel Publishing.

Acknowledgements

To begin, I would like to provide a land acknowledgement/Indigenous affirmation:

I am grateful and honoured to have written this book on the ancestral lands of the First Nation, Métis, and Inuit peoples. I am a settler of South Asian ancestry and I recognize that this book was written on the unceded territory of the Algonquin Anishinaabe Nation. I also acknowledge that the applicable treaties for this region are referred to as the Peace and Friendship Treaties. I reaffirm my responsibility to increase awareness and understanding of First Nations, Métis, and Inuit peoples and colonial legacy, and commit to strengthening my relationship with Indigenous peoples throughout Canada (Turtle Island).

Adapted from: www.uottawa.ca/about-us/indigenous/
indigenous-affirmation

Adding to this land acknowledgement/Indigenous affirmation, while attending relevant training about "*Incorporating Indigenous Peoples' Realities into our Courses,*" I learned that it is necessary to express gratitude for what is below our feet, the land we live on, the belief that we are all connected, and to respect the past and the future of this land that we reside upon. The notion of connection played a consistent role in the evolvement of this book. It truly requires a community of like-minded, visionary, and dedicated individuals to feel supported while writing a book of this magnitude. I am eternally grateful for everyone who was involved in the creation of this manuscript.

Thank you, Heather Evans, for your invaluable feedback on earlier drafts of this manuscript, and Julia Giordano, Pragati Sharma, and Jana Craddock, for later support on the final manuscript. Your editorial guidance and suggestions to enhance the existing manuscript are appreciated.

To Katy Reinhardt, my colleague and "local" editor, for editing this manuscript, offering invaluable recommendations and pep talks, being my wordsmith, and reminding both of us of our capacity. Thank you. This has been such an amazing journey, having you walk alongside and strengthen content for this timely book. I am forever appreciative for all the hours and work you put into this endeavour.

To Jean Ste-Amand, thank you for all your imaginative book framework transformations and patience during the editing process. You have a gift of bringing these visuals to life and give meaning within the manuscript text.

To my daughter Nadya, for your helpful feedback, research, and framework ideas. I am very fortunate to be able to collaborate and discuss these topics with you. Your future is so bright! Continue to shine and share your intelligence with everyone. Thanks to you and Ameya for feeling safe and comfortable disclosing how systemic oppression has impacted your lives. I am beyond proud of both of you and continue to learn from you.

To Steve, my partner, thank you for your patience. As you already know, writing this book required several late nights and endless manuscript revisions. I am in awe of your ability to quietly support my career-related adventures. I look forward to having more "free time" after the publication of this book so that we can just "be."

To my parents and SDK family for your unwavering support and love throughout my lifetime and beyond. Mom and Dad, some of my most notable writing occurred in your dining room, while I was in the deepest form of inner connection. I feel most safe, loved, and protected in your presence. Thank you for disclosing your trauma narratives, particularly regarding events that occurred during the 1947 Partition of India/Pakistan. These stories were immensely heart-wrenching yet informative in learning about our lineage's intergenerational trauma.

And lastly, to my BIPOC clients, students, colleagues, and friends who have endured different types of trauma; thank you for sharing your vulnerability and experiences. May you continue to encourage intergenerational healing and resilience.

Introduction to Trauma-Informed Psychotherapy for BIPOC Communities

Decolonizing Mental Health

"If you can't change reality, change your perceptions of it" declared Audre Lorde (1982, p. 18). Leaning into her profound words, how can we collectively deconstruct systemic racism and change the present sociopolitical narrative? Comparable to any trauma-informed initiative, this process starts at the grassroots level, in which we consider all ecosystems: home, academic setting, community, and host culture. Within these ecosystems, meaningful communication, relearning, as well as holding space by empathetic communities for individuals who are unable to commit to these changes are essential. Here is an example from my own narrative:

> More than a decade ago when my eldest daughter was in junior kindergarten, she asked me, "Mama, why did those girls call me spicy?" This inquiry is what categorically started discourse about racism in our home. I recall feeling saddened that she experienced racism at such a young age. We talked about the nuances associated with being spicy; she understood that these girls were clearly not able to articulate anything beyond her being spicy like Indian food. From that day onwards, instead of internalizing these racist comments, she became demonstrative, protective, and responsive about her cultural identity. In fact, with some cognitive reframing, my daughter became proud of her heritage and eager to educate others about her Punjabi-Sikh background.
>
> 10+ years later, after several transparent exchanges about culture, bullying, the patriarchy, capitalism, white supremacy, racism, and 2SLGBTQQIA+ rights, my daughters and I continue to have ad hoc conversations about these topics based on global events, Disney movies, and everything in between. My younger daughter expressed how the only black child in her culturally diverse classroom was being discriminated against. I decided to unpack this with her; she stated that these comments were based on the colour of his skin. I asked her who said this to him; she indicated two ethnic children (with lighter skin colour

DOI: 10.4324/9781003216568-1

profiles) made these remarks. She was bold enough to call these children out on their actions. She also informed her teacher who proceeded to remind these children about being respectful and inclusive towards everyone. These classmates apologized to this child; unfortunately, this incident was never discussed again. How could this common lived experience be incorporated into a grade school lesson plan or even as a teachable moment?

Our reflections about race and trauma eventually moved towards microaggressions in the workplace. Again, my eldest daughter revealed how uncomfortable she felt when residents at the long-term care facility would say "namaste" (a South Asian greeting, also commodified in Western yoga practices) or ask her, "Where are you really from?" based on their belief that she is South Asian. This dinnertime discussion evolved into conversation about whiteness, white supremacy, and related forms of oppression. Even as an immigrant child, I did not have dialogue of this nature with my first-generation parents. In fact, it was only during my adulthood that my parents disclosed their experiences of internalized/everyday racism which led to their suppressed symptoms associated with racial trauma.

Intergenerational trauma and trauma responses are interesting phenomena. In the instance of my eldest daughter, did trauma skip a generation, or are her trauma responses represented differently? My daughters are more aware of and vocal about racism and racial trauma; they internalize these experiences differently from how I did during my childhood (e.g., enabling teachers and peers to mispronounce my name by calling me "Paaavna"). After graduating from high school, I made a promise to myself to remind and educate individuals about how to pronounce my name. I also chose bicultural and pronounceable names for my daughters so that they would not tolerate these concealed microaggressions. Geneva Gay notes in her work about culturally responsive and inclusive teaching practices that trust needs to be established between an educator and student; part of this trust requires utmost respect for the student's cultural background, including how to say their names properly (Gay, 2002, 2018).

Discussions about trauma, systemic racism, and societal oppression embedded in white supremacy have continued to take place over the decades in sociopolitical milieus. More recently there has been an emphasis on creating space for rhetoric on such matters (e.g., race-based trauma and oppression). Focus has increased on the intersection between trauma, anti-racism, and mental health advocacy, which is crucial in decolonizing mental health within BIPOC (Black, Indigenous, and People of Colour) communities (Patel, 2015; Smith, 2012; Tuck & Yang, 2012). Current literature accentuates the need for practitioners to be culturally responsive and engage in cultural humility (Collins, 2018; Hook et al., 2013, 2017;

Lekas et al., 2020); however, the paradigm shift towards a more trauma-informed and anti-racist stance has not occurred.

While writing this book, the prevalence of racial oppression and hate crimes has increased and been amplified via social media. These prodigious events not only instill fear within BIPOC community members but also shape racialized and cultural psyches. It is disheartening that this suffering is perpetuated in various ecosystems. I constantly wonder what is NOT being discussed in either the home, academic setting, community, host culture, or as a whole. Why are individuals in the 2020s still thinking and reacting violently? How would my daughters respond now or in the future if a racist comment was said to them? This is one of the main reasons I have chosen to write about these concerns to further educate and dismantle systemic racism and preclude racial trauma at a young age.

What prevented change in the past? What has not worked in the past? The problem with all institutional systems is that they are trying to fill the colonial gap. The problem with all intuitional systems is the lack of BIPOC representation in the field. The problem with all intuitional systems is the lack of cultural humility and awareness. There is a need for systemic change and undoing of white supremacy, with severe repercussion if these parameters/rules are not met. No exceptions. How do we, as members of society, regain trust in others and the system?

Drawing from my clinical interactions with BIPOC clients, I became more cognizant of the emotional distress stemming from unresolved trauma. Trauma can result from birth order, sibling interactions, managing familial expectations, intergenerational conflict, and from one's culture being damaging. In some cultures, trauma and violence are normalized; an example is women treating women badly, which is intergenerational and acceptable in certain cultures. This may result in mental health diagnoses or coping strategies such as substance use to escape from recurring memories from the event(s) or simply to numb the existing associated feelings and thoughts. How long can one supress emotions regarding trauma? Reflection is imperative in therapy, regardless of one's support network. A therapist's objective worldview can be healing in and of itself and should subscribe to current culturally responsive and decolonized mental health approaches.

Intersectionality and Interest in This Topic

A tremendous amount of insight and learning was required to write this book. As such, I profoundly reflected upon my clinical, research, teaching, and lived experience. Likewise, I chose to complement my present knowledge by attending numerous social justice and trauma trainings and webinars. I read relevant and up-to-date literature to appreciate and refamiliarize my admiration for the implicit connection between current scholars and past ancestral theorists.

In accordance with self-reflexivity, I recognize my privilege and power in terms of my intersectionality and worldviews. I identify as a second-generation South Asian Punjabi-Sikh, heterosexual, able-bodied, neurodivergent, cisgender wounded healer female. Even though I was born and raised in Canada, I frequently justify and overexplain my birthplace as a second-generation settler, which I have learned can be a form of internalized racism (Houshmand et al., 2017; Pyke, 2010). I have overcome and pivoted these core values and beliefs, realizing they would be harmful in creating an authentic ethical space for my BIPOC clients. Other aspects of my intersectionality that have enhanced my privilege include being a mother, a child of educated voluntary immigrants, and having credentials and financial resources to be gainfully educated within a Canadian school system.

My education was very colonial and eurocentric, which I continue to unlearn and replace with more culturally responsive, trauma-informed practices. I believe that naming and checking in with my privilege was required throughout and beyond the production of this manuscript. By owning my intersectionality, I can identify and write as a racialized ally instead of a researcher, with hopes of barring a schism between these two aspects of my identity.

For over 20 years, I have provided psychotherapeutic services to BIPOC, immigrant, and 2SLGBTQQIA+ (two-spirit, lesbian, gay, bisexual, transgender, queer, questioning, intersex, asexual, and so forth) communities. My therapeutic approach is strongly rooted in intersectional feminism (Enns & Nutt Williams, 2012; hooks, 2014; Steinmetz, 2020) which, as defined by Kimberlé Crenshaw, is grounded in black feminist scholarship and consists of:

A lens, a prism, for seeing the way in which various forms of inequality often operate together and exacerbate each other. We tend to talk about race inequality as separate from inequality based on gender, class, sexuality or immigrant status. What's often missing is how some people are subject to all of these, and the experience is not just the sum of its parts.

(Crenshaw as cited in Steinmetz, 2020)

Interestingly, I was raised by two feminist-minded parents, who occasionally relented to the patriarchy due to the nature of South Asian culture. They were somehow conditioned to give in to older and archaic collectivist values.

Using this lens, I work with BIPOC clients and differentiate between several intersecting forms of oppression that contribute to their inner discord. Within a feminist perspective, I identify and consider the inclusivity of oppressed groups such as gender, race, ethnicity, sexual orientation, age, and class during therapeutic dialogue (Canadian Human Rights Act, 2021; Crenshaw, 2016; Evans et al., 2010). Many practitioners disregard the cultural aspect and fail to see colour in working with BIPOC clients; however, it emphatically plays a significant role in determining culturally responsive treatment planning, theoretical perspectives, and therapeutic approaches/strategies that are necessary to promote growth in our BIPOC clients. Self-disclosure, relating to and sharing lived experience with clients, and fostering an egalitarian rapport are some of the more eminent attributes of feminist theories (Seligman & Reichenberg, 2014).

I learn from clients in my practice who struggle and are affected by the psychological repercussions of racism and trauma-related events. Clients are eager to unpack their racist and traumatic experiences; as a psychotherapist, I understand the need to remain mindful of my personal biases, prejudices, and internalized oppression to demonstrate cultural empathy (Ridley & Lingle, 1996; Ridley & Shaw-Ridley, 2011), and to mirror these values to my BIPOC clients. As a wounded healer, a term first coined by Carl Jung in 1951, I can relate to and empathize with clients and recognize that healing can transpire in a non-linear manner (Dunning, 2006; Sedgwick, 2016; Smith, 2019). Western psychotherapeutic approaches are not always effective with BIPOC. With greater reason, culturally responsive therapists should actively listen to their BIPOC clients' narratives and consider offering decolonized practices such as fee reduction, accessible services, meeting the client where they are at, normalizing therapy, and not abiding to psychiatric labelling (Sodhi, 2021).

Throughout my career as a psychotherapist, I have listened to countless BIPOC narratives voicing present-day cultural ignorance, intergenerational trauma, and racism; these stories have left clients feeling unwelcome and alienated, which evolved into them feeling depressed or anxious based on their immigrant status and community membership. Referencing Dr. Thema Bryant-Davis' work (2019), as we shift from being culturally competent to anti-racist practitioners, how can we help BIPOC clients navigate systematic racism and societal oppression? How can we be more intentional with our clients, validate their emotions, demonstrate cultural humility, and hold space for their lived experience?

Part of the answer to these questions is the amplification of psychotherapeutic messaging that disputes our distorted perceptions of humanity. Thus, this book will highlight the connection between decolonizing psychotherapeutic practices via trauma-informed, anti-racist, anti-oppressive, and culturally responsive constructs. As culturally affirming and inclusive practitioners, integrating change, diversity, and inclusion within our clinical spaces is imperative. This goes beyond being woke – it is our role to raze the ecosystems that are bolstering oppression within our society and understand the impact it has on our clients' mindsets.

My research is anchored in social justice, critical race, and feminist principles and theories. For over 25 years, I have conducted research focussing on enhancing both awareness and respect towards multicultural populations, and I have built upon my initial curiosity surrounding various models of identity formation (Sodhi, 2017; Sodhi & Glickman, 2013). Since graduate school, I have learned that there is no shortage of multicultural research questions; there is, however, still a scarcity of literature about these much-needed topics, including content about culturally responsive trauma-informed practices.

Over the last decade, I have taught in a variety of post-secondary undergraduate and graduate settings. It is my intention in every course I teach to either include a cultural or decolonized component or both. I purposefully introduce material beneficial to working with multicultural demographics so that students can be more informed and educated about diverse cultures and develop racial stamina (DiAngelo, 2018; Gay, 2018). I have had success in presenting distinct cultural concepts to my students, and in return, they have expressed gratitude and the desire to become further culturally responsive.

Student feedback inspired me to write my first book: *Exploring Immigrant and Sexual Minority Mental Health: Reconsidering Multiculturalism* (Sodhi, 2017). Content from this book has been used to teach graduate-level counselling psychology courses. I shared a multimodal theoretical framework titled Diversity and Identity Formation Therapy (DIFT) to differentiate between theoretical orientations and strategies geared towards multicultural and 2SLGBTQQIA+ clients. I believe DIFT was a breakthrough in my students' appreciation that counselling is not standardized; being mindful of the client's cultural background and what approaches will resonate most with their therapeutic aspirations and visions is the essence of treatment planning.

On a personal note, I have deliberated upon my past narrative and now recognize my vulnerability regarding racism and trauma. I am very familiar with intergenerational and collective trauma. Both of my parents witnessed and survived the 1947 Partition of India/Pakistan. The colonization of language and culture via white infiltration during the British Rule continued when my parents immigrated to Canada, believing that speaking a eurocentric language would allow us, their offspring, to effortlessly assimilate into the host culture. My father also endured childhood trauma, which has been passed down in his academic and professional expectations for myself and my siblings. He believed in the importance of staying "cerebrally occupied" and to succeed; this may have been a trauma response (flight). I visited India multiple times throughout the

1980s during the height of Sikh genocide and terrorism. Based on our collective family history, I frequently question my somatic responses and what is possibly trapped within my nervous system. We all have therapeutic work to do, particularly unlearning familial expectations or internalized familial legacy burdens.

As a racialized immigrant child, I was not able to name everyday racism or even talk about these concerns with my family or ethnic friends until I was an adult. We did not discuss systems such as colonialism, the patriarchy, whiteness/white supremacy, capitalism, and individualism that were possibly normalized. Now as an adult, I am aware of how these past traumas informed my current mindset and ability to relate to BIPOC clients. I am facing forward, navigating resurfacing emotions, and sitting with and making space for the feelings associated with these events. I share more about these lived experience in the following chapters.

Definition of BIPOC, Trauma-Informed Therapy, and Decolonized Mental Health

Terminology

In this book, BIPOC refers to Black, Indigenous, and (other) People of Colour, or broadly to those demographics that are non-white. The term BIPOC first originated in 2013 on Twitter (Garcia, 2020), yet it was not until the Black Lives Matter (BLM) movement in 2020 that this term garnered further familiarity (Selvarajah et al., 2020). The breakdown of this acronym includes B (Black Americans/Canadians, African Caribbean/West Indian, or African, Black, Caribbean), I (Indigenous, Native Americans/Canadians; this book focuses on Canadian Indigenous groups), and POC (Asian, Pacific Islanders, South Asian, Latine/Hispanic, and Middle Eastern). The purpose of the BIPOC acronym is to support and mobilize intergroup solidarity, kindness, and compassion.

Generational status of BIPOC communities impacts intersectionality. First-generation immigrants are individuals born in their ancestral country; a 1.5-generation immigrant can be first-generation immigrant offspring who are also born in the ancestral country and immigrate with their parents between the ages of 7 and 17; second-generation immigrants are the offspring to first- or 1.5-generation immigrants; and third-generation immigrants are offspring to second-generation and so on (Sodhi, 2017; Thompson, 1974).

In working with BIPOC, migration patterns and diasporic experiences require exploration from therapists. This encompasses practitioners inquiring about the push factors (reasons for migrating such as poverty, lack of employment prospects, natural disasters, and sociopolitical fear) and pull factors (reasons not to migrate such as safety, educational and work opportunities, stability, better living standards) (Mohamed & Abdul-Talib, 2020). Therapists should also consider whether the client was a voluntary/involuntary immigrant or refugee, what the client's pre- and post-migration concerns were, and how ecosystems such as family, cultural/ethnic/racial community membership, and host culture perceptions influenced their intersectionality and cultural preservation/transmission. Lastly, therapists and clients alike should explore how mental health is either represented or hidden in the client's ancestral culture (e.g., is it denied, somaticized, or non-existent?) (Sodhi, 2021).

Trauma-informed practice has evolved over the last 30 years, and it will continue to progress and expand to encompass more inclusive approaches. Trauma-informed therapy requires becoming further aware of the client's background or past and curating a safe space by not retraumatizing the client (Sweeney et al., 2018). It consists of identifying the impact of the trauma on each client's brain, body, and existence, and then offering relevant trauma-informed interventions (e.g., polyvagal theory, somatic experiencing, EMDR) to work towards healing these aspects of their being (Dana, 2018; Levine, 1997; Shapiro, 2017). Substance Abuse and Mental Health Services (SAMHSA, 2014) posits that:

> A program, organization, or system that is trauma-informed *realizes* the widespread impact of trauma and understands potential paths for recovery; *recognizes* the signs and symptoms of trauma in clients, families, staff, and others involved with the system; and *responds* by fully integrating knowledge about trauma into policies, procedures, and practices, and seeks to actively resist re-traumatization.
>
> (p. 9)

Alongside these trauma-related concepts, trauma-informed therapy within my practice includes unpacking one's trauma narrative, considering how trauma is stored in the body using polyvagal methods, breaking intergenerational cycles, grieving and understanding personalized suffering, healing and resourcing inner confidence and resiliency, psychoeducation about trauma and the brain, inner child work/reparenting, naming trauma responses (e.g., fight, flight, freeze, or fawn), and developing applicable coping strategies (Dana, 2018, 2021; Stanley, 2019). Each of these topics are discussed throughout this book using decolonized language and philosophies.

There has been much attention regarding actively decolonizing mental health. The intent of this book is to inform and encourage readers to implement decolonized practices in their therapeutic, academic, and personal spaces. Steinman (2016) contends, "decolonization of the mind involves a fundamental emphasis on relationality – to ancestors, the natural world, other species, and more – against illusory individualizing, atomizing, and autonomous conceptions of selfhood and agency" (p. 229). We've reached a monumental era in which we cannot hide behind protective Western shields; in fact, we should confront and decentre these colonial, individualist, and white supremist barriers.

Decolonizing mental health is examined from trauma-informed, antiracist, anti-oppression, and culturally responsive standpoints in this book and is more elaborately analyzed in Part 4. To decolonize or deconstruct deeply entrenched Western vernacular, thoughts, and approaches, it is essential to use proper terminology, credit Eastern healing styles, and observe how Eastern and Western worldviews are internalized. When I teach diversity and multicultural counselling courses, I ask my students to consider language and messaging; for example, I request that they use the word "white" instead of "caucasian" as the latter may appear racist and dated (Moses, 2017).

Indigenizing curricula and offering culturally responsive viewpoints such as the inclusion of Indigenous voices (e.g., scholars, elders, or speakers), honouring oral traditions, and creating collaborative learning spaces are similarly being applied by educators (Gaudry & Lorenz, 2018). I prefer to offer the classroom configuration where seated desks are placed in a circular format, inviting a more egalitarian and inclusive learning space, resembling a healing circle. I choose this format rather than standing in the front of the class and providing lectures to the students. Students address me by my first name, instead of Dr. Sodhi, which also removes the academic hierarchy. These concepts will take time to become academically normalized, but every effort matters.

This book expands on inclusive and intersectional mental healthcare for BIPOC individuals. Such care requires being attentive to the client's intersectionality (e.g., culture, ethnicity, race, religion/faith, spirituality, language, gender, gender identity, social class, sexual orientation, ability, education, and age) and how this intersectionality informs therapy (Crenshaw, 1991). As therapists, we should meet the client where they are at in the therapeutic process, understanding and respecting the client's capacity to achieve therapeutic goals/intentions and tasks. Western diagnoses may be incongruent with what the client is experiencing; we must look beyond the physiological symptoms and examine systemic or root causes of their potential mental health condition, particularly if somatization is involved. Eloquently stated, decolonial therapists help clients "recognize their history, recover their ancestral memory, and critically understand their oppressive circumstances" (Comas-Díaz, 2021, p. 135).

Messaging concerning cultural competencies are evolving; establishing cultural responsivity and applying current language in our practice that will resonate with BIPOC is imperative to our growth as therapists. We must engage in cultural humility (Hook et al., 2017): recognize our biases and stereotypic beliefs, be culturally curious, self-reflect, and learn from our clients. The client is the expert of their narrative, and therapists honour and work with the client's expertise. Clients will teach the therapist about their life; yet, they should not teach us how to be culturally responsive.

There is a fine line between becoming a learner of the client's narrative and learning about their culture. Mental health professionals should be sufficiently informed that clients are not educating us or explaining their cultural backgrounds (Sodhi, 2017). There need to be preventative measures in place to preclude this shift in dynamics. Finally, clinicians need to establish a strong therapeutic alliance by means of collaborative therapeutic dialogue, conversation with a purpose, and shared language (Paré, 2013). As we support our BIPOC clients, speaking and understanding the same language, appreciating how oppressive systems impact their mental health, and learning to sit with a client who is experiencing trauma is necessary in cultivating a safe and trusting therapeutic atmosphere.

Purpose

I was inspired to write this book by conversations with BIPOC clients, students, family, friends, and colleagues. As issues such as intergenerational trauma, internalized racism, and systemic oppression are becoming increasingly ubiquitous within my clinical practice, the opportunity to share culturally responsive trauma-informed practices in the form of a book became enticing. I would build on my existing research in the field by communicating lived clinical and personal experience grounded in research specifically about trauma-informed therapy for BIPOC communities. Every contribution counts, and representation matters; there are not enough BIPOC therapists addressing and writing about the topics featured throughout this book.

The emergence of this book occurred at the beginning of the COVID-19 pandemic during a significant height of racial tension. The acronym BIPOC was becoming commonplace, and several sociopolitical movements came to the forefront. As we waited with bated breath for a vaccine, BIPOC communities continued to rally together for social and racial justice. A global effort to unlearn colonization, eurocentrism, white supremacy, and years of intergenerational oppression seemed to be rising. The collective trauma from a worldwide pandemic invited us all to create change in ourselves and others. In April 2021, I journalled the following in anticipation of writing this book:

What a week or so, starting with Vaisakhi (Sikh holiday) on April 13, trauma training on April 14, Sikh hate crime on April 15, decolonizing psychology training on April 16, George Floyd verdict on April 20, and a solidarity vigil on April 22. There is a sense of community, standing in solidarity to eradicate racial violence and educate the world about racial justice. Being a part of all these events over the span of nine days has demonstrated my yearning to be member of a consistent and productive allyship . . . and to write this much needed book for my BIPOC family worldwide. We stand alone and are bewildered; we stand together, and we are one with each other. We hold space and feel each other's pain which motivates us to make this a just world to thrive, instead of surviving. We should not be living in fear . . . even though, fear motivates change.

I have noticed throughout my lifetime that community care and learning about community formation are collaborative endeavours. A book can only educate you to a certain extent; it is important for therapists to consistently attend trainings and cultural events to capture all the attributes within the BIPOC community. It is a lifelong and collective learning process to decolonize mental health. We must migrate across borders to reinvent arbitrary rules, unlearn everything, build upon new learning, disrupt toxic oppressive cycles, and emanate as systemic therapists.

Who Is This Book For?

This book is primarily intended for current and future mental health professionals working directly with BIPOC individuals, especially if those professionals believe in multidisciplinary team/circle of care/community care and are interested in normalizing decolonized practices within their work space. This book can serve as a core resource for current and future psychologists, psychotherapists, social workers, supervisors within these mental health disciplines, community practitioners, and members of allied professions such as nurses, doctors, and lawyers.

Within this text, practitioners are reminded to assist clients in overcoming barriers to accessing counselling and help-seeking (Isaak et al., 2014); build culturally responsive and inclusive rapport (Sodhi, 2017; Sue & Sue, 2019); and gain a full understanding of each individual's cultural worldviews. I anticipate that by reading this book, therapists will be more capable of conceptualizing intersectionality and its impacts, structure sessions appropriately, and guide clients towards developing long-term and positive self-awareness. I hope to inspire mental health professionals to incorporate an anti-racist stance and provide therapy that honours intersectionality.

Grounded in trauma-informed perspectives (Bombay et al., 2009; Heart et al., 2011), intersectional theory (Crenshaw, 1989, 1991), and critical race theory (Bell, 1995; Delgado & Stefancic, 2017), this text encourages therapists to diversify their clinical approaches and further comprehend the unique considerations involved in working with BIPOC clients. The overarching purpose of this book is to expand upon this knowledge with existing language and messaging so that current mental health professionals can practice from a more trauma-informed and anti-racist platform.

I also hope that this book will motivate readers to reflect upon the evolution of trauma-informed practices over the last two decades. How is racism conceptualized and internalized? What happens when culture is deconstructed? Culture can affirm elements such as intersectionality, privilege, and power that can ultimately cause racism (overt and covert) and ignorance towards BIPOC communities. Anti-racist work will not only improve mental health services for BIPOC individuals but will mobilize communities, heighten social justice causes, and promote global healing. To quote Angela Davis (1983), "In a racist society it is not enough to be non-racist, we must be antiracist."

Presentation of Book

Given the current state of the world, the timing of this book is congruous. Early chapters offer psychoeducation and a theoretical overview of the above-mentioned constructs; case studies and narratives voiced by BIPOC individuals follow, and the book concludes with practical clinical interventions, future directions, and frameworks specifically for these communities. This book is therefore organized into the following five parts:

Part 1 – Dismantling and Understanding Trauma
Part 2 – Deconstructing Systemic Racism
Part 3 – Listening to Intergenerational BIPOC Narratives
Part 4 – Navigating Clinical Implications: Linking Theory to Practice
Part 5 – Concluding Thoughts and Offerings

Part 1 addresses dismantling and understanding trauma; it is comprised of three chapters. Chapter 1 defines and names trauma, Chapter 2 imparts myths and types of trauma, and Chapter 3 outlines culturally responsive trauma-informed psychotherapy. Discourse pertaining to trauma continues to exist beyond post-traumatic stress disorder. For immigrants, it can involve migratory, colonial, intergenerational, intersectional, and systemic trauma (Bombay et al., 2009; Fast & Collin-Vézina, 2010; Sodhi, 2017). Trauma among BIPOC may also arise as race-based traumatic stress, racialized trauma, developmental trauma, collective trauma, and cultural trauma (Alexander, 2016; Comas-Díaz et al., 2019; Maté & Maté, 2022).

The existence of various forms of trauma as well as an understanding of Eastern approaches to assist BIPOC in healing from trauma are two constructs that modern rhetoric fails to address (Sodhi, 2022; van der Kolk, 2014). Moreover, emphasis on colonial methods and neurology in the *Diagnostic and Statistical Manual of Mental Disorders* (DSM-5) lend to more Western therapeutic strategies. The first part of the chapter conveys knowledge and theory about naming traumatic events; the manifestations of trauma; how the brain and body store trauma; and strategies to break intergenerational trauma cycles (Perry & Winfrey, 2021; Fisher, 2017). A table representing different types of trauma is provided and discussed.

Part 2 deconstructs systemic racism and consists of three chapters. Chapter 4 conceptualizes racism; Chapter 5 identifies the levels, forms, and movements of racism; and Chapter 6 highlights mental health implications and developing an anti-racist stance. Together, these chapters link theoretical concepts such as critical race theory; the history of oppression (Freire, 1970); intersectionality; origins of structural and systemic racism; capitalism, colonialism, and the patriarchy; internalized racism; racial gaslighting; interminority racism; white supremacy; white privilege; naming one's white fragility and white guilt; the impact of colonialism within a global context; and latent racism, shadeism, and colourism (Bhopal, 2018; Constantine, 2007).

Rooted in Harro's cycle of socialization framework (2000), Part 2 also explores past and current sociopolitical movements, including but not limited to *Black Lives Matter*, Indigenous rights, Islamophobia, Sikhphobia, anti-Asian racism (especially since the beginning of the COVID-19 pandemic), cancel culture, and boycotting national holidays (i.e., Canada Day/July 4th), and culminates with insight about the need for land acknowledgements, anti-racist practices, racial justice, consistent allyship (productive versus performative), and solidarity.

Part 3 contextualizes intergenerational BIPOC narratives from members of the Black, Indigenous, South Asian, Latine, and Asian communities. These narratives include traumatic, racial, and oppressive content from Parts 1 and 2 and function as case studies for the case conceptualizations and interventions in Part 4.

Part 4 discusses navigating clinical implications and linking theory to practice; it is divided into three chapters. Chapter 7 communicates decolonizing mental health practices, Chapter 8 describes a trauma-informed integrated model and introduces inclusion and healing therapy (IHT), and Chapter 9 revisits BIPOC narratives from Part 3. As we collectively raise awareness toward anti-racist causes, it is important to apply relevant decolonized approaches within our clinical practices as therapists.

Referencing the constructs examined in Parts 1 and 2, this part of the text sheds light on anti-oppressive mental health practices; overcoming barriers to and cultural stigmas about accessing care and mitigating withdrawal from mental health services; educating BIPOC regarding mental health and healing (Sodhi, 2017; Sue, 2001); and strategies to eradicate internalized racism. The narratives from Part 3 are analyzed (unpacked) in this section through case conceptualizations, treatment plans, and exercises to exemplify how to effectively work with BIPOC clients.

Part 5 of the book aims to apply theory into practice, or "unlearning and relearning." It underscores both the meaning of shifting from being culturally competent to trauma-informed and anti-racist practitioners, as well as the importance of decolonizing therapy classrooms and academic curricula via culturally responsive practices and trauma-informed pedagogy (Gay, 2018; Reyes et al., 2021; Singh et al., 2020). Drawing from liberation psychology (Martín-Baró, 1996) and Harro's cycle of liberation (2000), IHT equips clients with culturally responsive strategies for how to reframe trauma responses, actualize intergenerational resilience, and embody healing through community and self-care practices.

There is debate about whether the theoretical approaches and interventions outlined in this book are actually culturally responsive; such colloquy is embedded in misinformation and ignorance about the complexities intrinsic to BIPOC cases, barriers that BIPOC face, and fundamental misunderstandings about somatization. One must include anti-racist, anti-oppressive, feminist, social justice, and culturally responsive modalities (Sodhi, 2021). As Tuck and Yang (2012) affirmed, "decolonization is not a metaphor. When metaphor invades decolonization, it kills the very possibility of decolonization" (p. 3). There have been numerous efforts to support decolonized practices in our therapeutic settings. I would like to break down silos between therapists, stand together in solidarity, and dismantle the colonialist ways to normalize trauma-informed practices for BIPOC communities.

References

Alexander, J. C. (2016). Culture trauma, morality and solidarity: The social construction of "Holocaust" and other mass murders. *Thesis Eleven, 132*, 3–16.

Bell, D. (1995). Who's afraid of critical race theory? *University of Illinois Law Review, 4*, 893–910.

Bhopal, K. (2018). *White privilege: The myth of a post-racial society*. Policy Press.

Bombay, A., Matheson, K., & Anisman, H. (2009). Intergenerational trauma: Convergence of multiple processes among First Nations peoples in Canada. *International Journal of Indigenous Health, 5*(3), 6–47.

Bryant-Davis, T. (Ed.). (2019). *Multicultural feminist therapy: Helping adolescent girls of color to thrive*. American Psychological Association.

Canadian Human Rights Act. (2021). *(R.S.C., 1985, c. H-6)*. Retrieved August 27, 2021, from https://canlii.ca/t/555n8

Collins, S. (2018). *Embracing cultural responsivity and social justice: Re-shaping professional identity in counselling psychology*. Counselling Concepts.

Comas-Díaz, L. (2021). Sociopolitical trauma: Ethnicity, race, and migration. In P. Tummala- Narra (Ed.), *Trauma and racial minority immigrants: Turmoil, uncertainty, and resistance* (pp. 127–146). American Psychological Association.

Comas-Díaz, L., Hall, G. N., & Neville, H. A. (2019). Racial trauma: Theory, research, and healing: Introduction to the special issue. *American Psychologist, 74*(1), 1–5.

Constantine, M. G. (2007). Racial microaggressions against African American clients in cross-racial counseling relationships. *Journal of Counseling Psychology, 54*, 1–16.

Crenshaw, K. (1989). Demarginalizing the intersection of race and sex: A black feminist critique of antidiscrimination doctrine, feminist theory and antiracist politics. *University of Chicago Legal Forum, 1989*(1), 139.

Crenshaw, K. (1991). Mapping the margins: Intersectionality, identity politics, and violence against women of color. *Stanford Law Review, 43*(6), 1241–1299.

Crenshaw, K. (2016, October). The urgency of intersectionality. [Video]. *Ted-Women*. Kimberlé Crenshaw: The urgency of intersectionality | TED Talk.

Dana, D. (2018). *The polyvagal theory in therapy: Engaging the rhythm of regulation*. W.W. Norton.

Dana, D. (2021). *Anchored: How to befriend your nervous system using polyvagal theory*. Sound True.

Davis, A. Y. (1983). *Women, race & class*. Vintage Books.

Delgado, D., & Stefancic, J. (2017). *Critical race theory: An introduction* (3rd ed.). NYU Press.

DiAngelo, R. (2018). *White fragility: Why it's so hard for white people to talk about racism*. Beacon Press.

Dunning, T. (2006). Caring for the wounded healer – nurturing the self. *Journal of Bodywork and Movement Therapies, 10*(4), 251–260.

Enns, C. Z., & Nutt Williams, E. (2012). *The Oxford handbook of feminist counseling psychology*. Oxford University Press.

Evans, K. M., Kincade, E. A., & Seem, S. R. (2010). *Introduction to feminist therapy: Strategies for social and individual change*. Sage Publications.

Fast, E., & Collin-Vézina, D. (2010). Historical trauma, race-based trauma, and resilience of Indigenous peoples: A literature review. *First Peoples Child & Family Review, 5*(1), 126–136.

Fisher, J. (2017). *Healing the fragmented selves of trauma survivors: Overcoming internal self-alienation*. Routledge.

Freire, P. (1970). *Pedagogy of the oppressed*. Continuum International.

Garcia, S. E. (2020). *Where did BIPOC come from?* Retrieved January 16, 2022, from www.nytimes.com/article/what-is-bipoc.html

Gaudry, A., & Lorenz, D. (2018). Indigenization as inclusion, reconciliation, and decolonization: Navigating the different versions for Indigenizing the Canadian academy. *AlterNative: An International Journal of Indigenous Peoples, 14*(3), 218–227.

Gay, G. (2002). Preparing culturally responsive teaching. *Journal of Teacher Education, 53*, 106–116.

Gay, G. (2018). *Culturally responsive teaching: Theory, research and practice* (3rd ed.). Teachers College Press.

Harro, B. (2000). The cycle of liberation. In M. Adams, W. Blumenfeld, R. Castaneda, H. Hackman, M. Peters & X. Zuniga (Eds.), *Readings for diversity and social justice* (pp. 463–469). Routledge.

Harro, B. (2000). The cycle of socialization. In M. Adams, W. Blumenfeld, R. Castaneda, H. Hackman, M. Peters & X. Zuniga (Eds.), *Readings for diversity and social justice* (pp. 15–20). Routledge.

Heart, M. Y., Chase, J., Elkins, J., & Altschul, D. B. (2011). Historical trauma among Indigenous Peoples of the Americas: Concepts, research, and clinical considerations. *Journal of Psychoactive Drugs, 43*(4), 282–290.

Hook, J. N., Davis, D. E., Owen, J., Worthington, E. L. Jr., & Utsey, S. O. (2013). Cultural humility: Measuring openness to culturally diverse clients. *Journal of Counseling Psychology, 60*(3), 353–366.

Hook, J. N., Don, D., Owen, J., & DeBlaere, C. (2017). *Cultural humility: Engaging diverse identities in therapy* (pp. 43–64). American Psychological Association.

hooks, b. (2014). Visionary feminism. In *Feminism is for everybody* (2nd ed.). Routledge.

Houshmand, S., Spanierman, L. B., & De Stephano, J. (2017). Racial microaggressions: A primer with implications for counseling practice. *International Journal of Advanced Counselling, 39*, 203–216.

Isaak, C. A., Mota, N., Medved, M., Katz, L. Y., Elias, B., Mignone, J., Munro, G., Kirmayer, L. J., Gone, J. P., & Moses, J. (2014). Rethinking historical trauma. *Transcultural Psychiatry, 51*(3), 299–319.

Lekas, H.-M., Pahl, K., & Fuller Lewis, C. (2020). Rethinking cultural competence: Shifting to cultural humility. *Health Services Insights*, 1–4.

Levine, P. A. (1997). *Waking the tiger: Healing trauma.* North Atlantic Books.

Lorde, A. (1982). *Zami: A new spelling of my name.* Crossing Press.

Martín-Baró, I. (1996). *Writings for a liberation psychology.* Harvard University Press.

Maté, G., & Maté, D. (2022). *The myth of normal: Trauma, illness, and healing in a toxic culture.* Knopf Canada.

Mohamed, M.-A., & Abdul-Talib, A.-N. (2020). Push-pull factors influencing international return migration intentions: A systematic literature review. *Journal of Enterprising Communities: People and Places in the Global Economy, 14*(2), 231–246.

Moses, Y. (2017). *Why do we keep using the word "caucasian"?* Retrieved January 22, 2022, from www.sapiens.org/column/race/caucasian-terminology-origin/

Paré, D. A. (2013). *The practice of collaborative counselling and psychotherapy: Developing skills in culturally mindful helping.* Sage Publications.

Patel, L. (2015). *Decolonizing educational research: From ownership to answerability* (1st ed.). Routledge.

Perry, B., & Winfrey, O. (2021). *What happened to you?* Flatiron Books.

Pyke, K. D. (2010). What is internalized racial oppression and why don't we study it? Acknowledging racism's hidden injuries. *Sociological Perspectives, 53*(4), 551–572.

Reyes, V., Clancy, S., Koge, H., Richardson, K., & Taylor, P. (2021). Decolonising globalised curriculum landscapes: The identity and agency of academics. *London Review of Education, 19*(1), 26, 1–13.

Ridley, C. R., & Lingle, D. W. (1996). Cultural empathy in multicultural counseling: A multidimensional process model. In P. Pedersen, J. Draguns, W. Lonner & J. Trimble (Eds.), *Counseling across cultures* (4th ed., pp. 21–46). Sage.

Ridley, C. R., & Shaw-Ridley, M. (2011). Multicultural counseling competencies: An analysis of research on clients' perceptions. *Journal of Counseling Psychology*, *58*, 16–21.

Sedgwick, D. (2016). *The wounded healer: Countertransference from a Jungian perspective*. Routledge.

Seligman, L., & Reichenberg, L. W. (2014). *Theories of counseling and psychotherapy: Systems, strategies, and skills*. Pearson Education.

Selvarajah, S., Deivanayagam, T. A., Lasco, G., Scafe, S., White, A., Zembe-Mkabile, W., & Devakumar, D. (2020). Categorisation and minoritisation. *BMJ Global Health*, *5*(12), e004508, 1–4.

Shapiro, F. (2017). *Eye movement desensitization and reprocessing (EMDR) therapy: Basic principles, protocols and procedures* (3rd ed.). Guilford Press.

Singh, A. A., Appling, B., & Trepal, H. (2020). Using the multicultural and social justice counseling competencies to decolonize counseling practice: The important roles of theory, power, and action. *Journal of Counseling and Development*, *98*, 261–271.

Smith, L. T. (2012). *Decolonizing methodologies: Research and Indigenous peoples* (2nd ed.). Zedd Books.

Smith, M. (2019). Wounding healers. Killing with kindness on the road to hell. *Journal of Social Work Practice*, *33*(1), 109–115.

Sodhi, P. K. (2017). *Exploring immigrant and sexual minority mental health: Reconsidering multiculturalism*. Routledge.

Sodhi, P. K. (2021). Decolonizing psychotherapeutic practices for BIPOC clients. Webinar hosted by the *Canadian Counselling and Psychotherapy Association*, October 27, 2021.

Sodhi, P. K. (2022). Trauma-informed care for BIPOC communities. Speaker series hosted by the *Canadian Counselling and Psychotherapy Association*, November 16, 2022.

Sodhi, P. K., & Glickman, D. (2013). Sexual minorities: Exploring the sexual identity development and ethnic identity formation of multicultural populations. Paper presented at the *Canadian Counselling and Psychotherapy Association inaugural research conference*, Ottawa, Ontario, February 16–17, 2013.

Stanley, E. A. (2019). *Widen the window: Training your brain and body to thrive during stress and recover from trauma*. Avery.

Steinman, E. W. (2016). Decolonization not inclusion: Indigenous resistance to American settler colonialism. *Sociology of Race and Ethnicity*, *2*(2), 219–236.

Steinmetz, K. (2020). *She coined that term 'intersectionality' over 30 years ago. Here's what it means to her today*. Retrieved January 13, 2022, from https://time.com/5786710/kimberle-crenshaw-intersectionality/

Substance Abuse and Mental Health Services Administration (SAMHSA). (2014). *SAMHSA's concept of trauma and guidance for a trauma-informed approach*. Substance Abuse and Mental Health Services Administration.

Sue, D. W. (2001). Multidimensional facets of cultural competence. *The Counseling Psychologist*, *29*, 790–821.

Sue, D. W., & Sue, D. (2019). *Counseling the culturally diverse: Theory and practice* (8th ed.). John Wiley & Sons, Inc.

Sweeney, A., Filson, B., Kennedy, A., Collinson, L., & Gillard, S. (2018). A paradigm shift: Relationships in trauma-informed mental health services. *Bjpsych Advances*, *24*, 319–333.

Thompson, M. (1974). The second generation: Punjabi or English? *New Community*, *3*(3), 242–248.

Tuck, E., & Yang, W. K. (2012). Decolonization is not a metaphor. *Decolonization: Indigeneity, Education & Society*, *1*(1), 1–40.

van der Kolk, B. A. (2014). *The body keeps the score: Brain, mind, and body in the healing of trauma*. Viking.

Part 1

Dismantling and Understanding Trauma

Introduction

Admittedly, this was the hardest part of the book to write as I reflect upon my personal trauma, my clients' narratives, and research topics about this subject matter. As a child, I journalled about my life and travels, as I do present-day. I have always found it grounding; however, writing about trauma elicited somatic responses that were likely stored in my nervous system for several years. This introspection yielded numerous follow-up questions about my ancestors and much needed intergenerational healing.

Currently in trauma-informed literature, there has been a shift from judgement to concern by reframing "What is wrong with you?" to "What happened to you?" (Maté & Maté, 2022; Perry & Winfrey, 2021). Theorists are trying to understand the inner workings of internalized trauma and how it affects one's present-day thoughts, feelings, and behaviours. This part of the book elucidates what trauma is and how it exists in all of our lives; we all have trauma imprints from the past. Even within my narrative, I am re-evaluating different types of traumas endured throughout my lifetime and how my trauma responses towards these events have been minimized.

Trauma has countless sources, each of which can cause disconnection within ourselves; trauma is not limited to a war, pandemic, systemic oppression, religious persecution, or scarcity. For some BIPOC, events may not be as traumatic and may be normalized. Normalizing culturally related trauma does not mean it did not exist; it just needs to be unpacked and further deliberated. It is only retrospectively after a trauma when we start to question how our nervous system responds/reacts to certain situations that we become aware of the trauma that is either trapped in our bodies or embedded in our memories. Trauma does not discriminate and can present as shame, depression, exhaustion, insomnia, and more. Cycles may perpetuate (e.g., not dealt with, ignored, and passed on) due to barriers that are discussed shortly or by means of spiritual

DOI: 10.4324/9781003216568-2

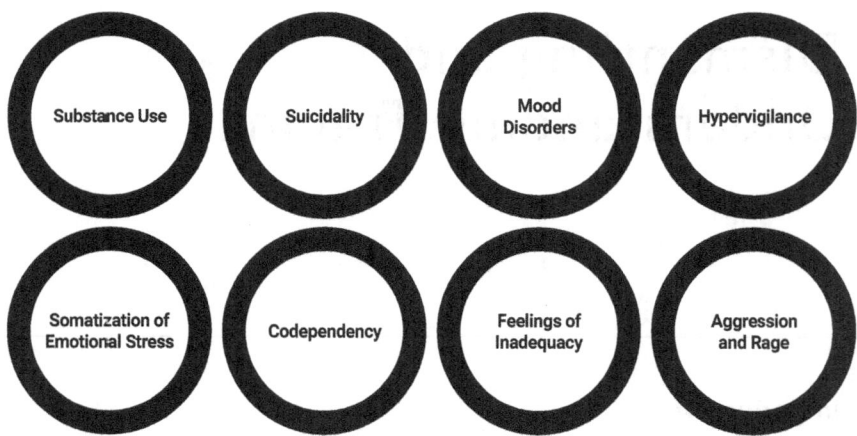

Figure 1.1 The impact of trauma within BIPOC communities

bypassing (e.g., turning to faith instead of processing trauma). Unlearning trauma equals breaking cycles plus conscious healing. Culturally responsive trauma-informed therapy requires that the healing process restores safety, reconnects us to ourselves, and removes the othering so that BIPOC can heal together.

While writing this book, I was reminded daily of how trauma has established itself in my clients' lives. BIPOC communities confront trauma via migratory hardships, white supremacy, capitalism, systemic racism and hate crimes, the patriarchy, a lack of identity or sense of belonging, intergenerational trauma, and colonial oppression. As a BIPOC woman, I have drawn from my lived experience to help clients understand and heal from these past traumas. This has been a collaborative process of being able to engage in self-compassion, name events, and unlearn internalized traits that have been brought on by varied forms of trauma. With further dialogue and awareness in the therapeutic space, clients will be able to break intergenerational cycles and ultimately actualize healing.

Most of us have experienced some form of trauma or suffering during our lifetime, whether we are able to name it or even have the language to articulate what exactly happened. Part of the undertaking in writing this book is to invite other BIPOC to reflect upon the trauma they may have either bypassed or denied in the past. It is quite the exercise and can leave one feeling activated within their nervous system. Trauma can be perceived in different contexts. For some individuals, trauma can be obvious and acute. Others might normalize the trauma, believing it was a part of their life that happened for a reason. As I continue to write this book, I am in awe of the number of trauma survivors I not only counsel but admire from afar.

In the spirit of being transparent and connected to this topic, my trauma narrative is the following:

Over the past seven years, while working alongside my spiritual therapist, I have taken monumental steps towards understanding my trauma narrative. One could say it started with the trauma my maternal grandmother encountered bearing seven daughters, and no sons. Thankfully, this patriarchal belief that males are better than females was debunked by my progressive maternal grandfather who refused to have a second wife to bear a male child. Sadly, even this option resulted in my grandmother feeling inferior and not good enough for my grandfather.

My grandmother's core beliefs about unworthiness were compounded by what transpired during the 1947 Partition of India/Pakistan when my grandparents fled Pakistan and migrated to India. Upon my visits to India, I witnessed first hand the effect of the country's history on my grandmother, who would attentively lock and check the doors of the kothi (house) to ensure we were all safe inside. At this point, she was walking with a cane and would use the bottom part of her cane to maneuver the upper locks of the doors. During my childhood, I thought she had a wonderful system, but now, I realize it was more of a ritual brought on by intrusive thoughts of not feeling safe. This "ritual" has been passed down to my mother, and myself, who constantly check if doors are locked . . . This was the beginning of intergenerational trauma that was not really spoken of until recently and instead normalized. Perhaps there was a stigma associated with being anxious or afraid or even believing a situation is traumatic. Yet this led to me developing all forms of subjugation (people pleasing), perfectionism, and feelings of inadequacy.

I was raised in Halifax, Nova Scotia, where most of the South Asian community at the time was educated and had secure employment. The immigrant dream was in full effect, and again, from my previous research, an immigrant's success is strongly determined by their children's career trajectories (Sodhi, 2002). Both of my parents are highly accomplished, with education from India and Canada, and landed permanent employment as educators and psychologists in Nova Scotia. There was a strong emphasis in our home to be educated and financially independent, another transgenerational trait. I recall being told by my fourth-grade teacher that I was not smart enough, and I would never graduate from high school. This was the first of many educational events that hampered my self-confidence. In university, my siblings both pursued science-related degrees. I attempted a degree in commerce but eventually appreciated that my interest was more in psychology and education. Unfortunately, I carried these inadequacies with me during my schooling, feeling that I needed to prove myself more to the community, and therefore completed four degrees: B.A., B.Ed., M.Ed., and Ed.D. Several years later, one of my closest friends said that I essentially pushed boundaries and barriers by choosing a career path based on my passions instead of community expectations.

Another community characteristic involved backhanded shaming and gaslighting, whether it was about body image, marriage, career choices, or overall success. I was told by one community "Aunty" to go on a diet at the age of 11 and by another "Aunty" who said that if I do not get married by age 27, I will not get married at all. Again, I internalized these comments that intensified my already prominent feelings of low self-worth. In fact, I have body image issues and body dysmorphia to this day, and always aspire to be healthy and fit. I dealt with unresolved bullying and body image issues throughout my schooling, where I was not seen or heard. I am frequently reminded of these memories.

This distorted self-perception led to a 14+ year marriage to a South Asian man who was emotionally, financially, and verbally abusive towards me. I was engaged to him for eight months and felt pressured to get married due to previous community shaming. While dating, I truly believed that he would change, our relationship would become stronger, we would have better communication, and live a long and happy married life. I tried for innumerable years to make the marriage work, as I strongly believed in a cohesive family unit and only wanted the best for our children. It became worse as his older sister started to further undermine, gaslight, emotionally admonish, and exclude me from their family dynamic. My separation from him served as a form of intergenerational healing. I was a cycle breaker of sorts, being the first in my family to leave a toxic marriage.

It has been challenging sharing my vulnerability regarding trauma and shame, and the impact trauma can have on one's physical and mental health. I feared professional and community stigma. I invested a tremendous amount in my career and research to cope with all the marital tension. I asserted myself, established boundaries, and persevered for the sake of my children. I initially developed heightened anxiety and panic attacks but then all this unresolved trauma created cardiac issues and finally a cancer diagnosis. For the longest time, I did not share my diagnosis with professional colleagues due to shame, judgment, and implicit biases. I was also protecting my vulnerability throughout this process and did not allow my physical health issues to become a part of my intersectionality.

These health conditions have since been resolved; however, during this precarious time, and particularly when I met with cardiologists and oncologists, I trauma responded and remained in flight mode throughout the whole "detour," as I still refuse to call it a journey. I kept busy with self-development, my clinical practice, teaching, and the final stages of the publication of my first book; these activities were not supported by my doctors. I was told that if I did not follow recommended standard of care, I would die and never see my daughters grow up. There was a significant amount of fear mongering, but I stood my ground and was able to negotiate a treatment plan that would offer optimal results and long-term health. I chose to be realistic with my separated marital status, being a single parent, and rebuilding my career. In the end, everything worked out, with ancestral guidance from my matriarch, a wonderful support network, and a team of decolonial healers.

In terms of intergenerational healing, I praise my parents who seamlessly modeled resiliency after attending to their own serious health issues. They were able to author books, participate in community care, practice yoga, enjoy gardening, and demonstrate altruistic acts (seva) of loving kindness (metta) as part of their healing journey. They have taught me that anything is possible, regardless of the traumas we experience. When I slip into these old thought patterns, I engage in more gratitude practices and learn to fall in love with myself again. I tune into wellness revelations, where I listen to and respect my body and inner capacity. I share this narrative, as I notice similar trends with my BIPOC clients. There are noteworthy, interconnected links between trauma, stress, physical, and mental health that cannot be denied or overlooked (Maté, 2004). I am hoping that my traumatic experiences and how the accumulation of trauma (in one's nervous system) can impact their physical wellbeing will help readers of this book.

Everything considered, it is imperative to fathom the origins of trauma-informed care and what "trauma-informed integrative approach" means. Trauma-informed care is a combination of inclusivity, equity, and intersectionality while simultaneously upholding physical and emotional safety, security, stability, and trust for individuals who have experienced trauma and are trying to achieve agency and recovery from events (Substance Abuse and Mental Health Services Administration, 2014). Trauma-informed training teaches practitioners about the following constructs and best practices: the types of trauma; somatic aspects (mind-body connection); trauma responses, including emotional and nervous system regulation (self-regulate and co-regulate); reframing, safety, stabilization, and grounding techniques; internal and community resources; and collective and community care practices. The intention here is to preclude individuals from being retraumatized, and rather feel supported and heard to recover from these events (Sweeney et al., 2018).

These six pillars are a hybrid of the core values of trauma-informed care discussed by Fallot and Harris (2001, 2009) and the Substance Abuse and Mental Health Services Administration (2014):

1. **Safety:** create a physical, social, gender, emotional, cultural, and psychological safe space for individuals.
2. **Trustworthiness and transparency:** a non-judgmental, respectful, and predictable backdrop that facilitates building trust and authenticity.
3. **Peer support:** cultivate a sense of belonging supported by like-minded individuals.
4. **Collaboration and mutuality:** eradicate power dynamics and instead validate decision-making processes.
5. **Empowerment, voice, and choice:** foster agency and heightened awareness regarding resources to encourage inner strength, healing, and resilience.
6. **Cultural, historical, and gender issues:** overcome biases, promote inclusivity, and openly discuss intersectional and trauma-related concerns.

Guarino et al. (2009) impart a trauma-informed organizational self-assessment comprised of eight culturally responsive principles:

1. Understanding Trauma and Its Impact
2. Promoting Safety
3. Ensuring Cultural Competencies
4. Supporting Consumer Control, Choice, and Autonomy
5. Sharing Power and Governance
6. Integrating Care
7. Healing Happens in Relationships
8. Recovery Is Possible

These guiding principles support BIPOC to feel supported by:

> Understanding how cultural context influences one's perception of and response to traumatic events and the recovery process; respecting diversity within the program, providing opportunities for consumers to engage in cultural rituals, and using interventions respectful of and specific to cultural backgrounds.
>
> (Guarino et al., 2009, p. 17)

As well as endorsing a holistic and community care approach that fundamentally advances safety, healing, and resiliency.

Within our work with BIPOC, there is the inevitability of creating a trauma-informed community and realizing the potential impact it might have on individual, familial, community, and societal systems (Shramko et al., 2019). This might involve building a community whose motivation is to sustain resiliency from members of different intersectional, academic, familial, and societal systems (Matlin et al., 2019). Concurrently,

> participating communities in these initiatives may provide training in resilience and trauma awareness to community stakeholders, establish trauma-informed service networks, share tips and resources for community development and coalition building, infuse community settings with the principles of trauma-informed practice, and advocate for specific trauma-responsive policies.
>
> (Substance Abuse and Mental Health Services
> Administration, 2014, as cited in
> Matlin et al., 2019, p. 2)

For these interventions to produce long-term results, consistent and purposeful communication needs to occur between productive communities and their like-minded members.

I respect my BIPOC clients for their intergenerational resiliency and capacity to contend with stressful situations, particularly with no privilege or *free passes* provided. In some ways, trauma can make a person stronger and more resourceful in terms of encountering future traumatic events. I believe this is at the core of intergenerational resilience. The next three chapters elaborate upon what trauma entails, its diverse forms of presentation, and culturally responsive strategies to manage personalized trauma.

References

Fallot, R., & Harris, M. (2009). *Creating cultures of trauma-informed care (CCTIC): A self-assessment and planning protocol*. Retrieved January 25, 2023, from www.healthcare.uiowa.edu/icmh/documents/CCTICSelf-Assessmentand PlanningProtocol0709.pdf

Guarino, K., Soares, P., Konnath, K., Clervil, R., & Bassuk, E. (2009). *Trauma-informed organizational toolkit*. Center for Mental Health Services, Substance Abuse and Mental Health Services Administration. Retrieved January 25, 2023, from www.air.org/sites/default/files/downloads/report/Trauma-Informed_Organizational_Toolkit_0.pdf

Harris, M. E., & Fallot, R. D. (2001). *Using trauma theory to design service systems*. Jossey-Bass.

Maté, G. (2004). *When the body says no: The cost of hidden stress*. Vintage Canada.

Maté, G., & Maté, D. (2022). *The myth of normal: Trauma, illness, and healing in a toxic culture*. Knopf Canada.

Matlin, S. L., Champine, R. B., Strambler, M. J., O'Brien, C., Hoffman, E., Whitson, M., Kolka, L., & Tebes, J. K. (2019). A community's response to adverse childhood experiences: Building a resilient, trauma-informed community. *American Journal of Community Psychology, 64*(3–4), 451–466.

Perry, B., & Winfrey, O. (2021). *What happened to you?* Flatiron Books.

Shramko, M., Pfluger, L., & Harrison, B. (2019). *Intersectionality and trauma-informed application for maternal and child health research and evaluation: An initial summary of the literature* [Unpublished Manuscript]. Minnesota Department of Health.

Sodhi, P. (2002). *Punjabi women living in Eastern Canada: A study exploring parental attitudes, intergenerational cultural preservation, and ethnic identity formation* [Unpublished Doctoral Dissertation, The Ontario Institute for Studies in Education of the University of Toronto].

Substance Abuse and Mental Health Services Administration (SAMHSA). (2014). *SAMHSA's concept of trauma and guidance for a trauma-informed approach (HHS Publication No. SMA 14–4884)*. Substance Abuse and Mental Health Services Administration.

Sweeney, A., Filson, B., Kennedy, A., Collinson, L., & Gillard, S. (2018). A paradigm shift: Relationships in trauma-informed mental health services. *BJPsych Advances, 24*(5), 319–333.

Chapter 1

Defining and Naming Trauma

This chapter offers an in-depth perspective on trauma, including defining trauma through a BIPOC lens. Etymologically, the word "trauma" is derived from the Greek term for "wound," which can encompass myriad long- and short-term physical, emotional, biological, and psychological symptoms as well as one's identity formation and social interactions. Definitions, events, experiences, effects, and trauma and the brain are specified in the following passages.

Definitions

Trauma has evolved over the last 30 years to include events beyond wars, childhood trauma, and natural disasters. Thankfully, in the recent past, individuals have been coming to terms with their trauma and now appear more open to talking about what happened to them. Trauma can surface in a variety of ways and can be strongly linked to one's mental health. Noted in the next section are a selection of trauma-related definitions:

According to the American Psychiatric Association's *Diagnostic and Statistical Manual of Mental Disorders*, trauma can be:

> Exposure to actual or threatened death, serious injury, or sexual violence in one (or more) of the following ways: directly experiencing the traumatic event(s); witnessing, in person, the traumatic event(s) as it occurred to others; learning that the traumatic event(s) occurred to a close family member or close friend (in case of actual or threatened death of a family member or friend, the event(s) must have been violent or accidental); or experiencing repeated or extreme exposure to aversive details of the traumatic event(s).
>
> (APA, 2013)

DOI: 10.4324/9781003216568-3

The American Psychological Association suggests:

> Trauma is an emotional response to a terrible event like an accident, rape, or natural disaster. Immediately after the event, shock and denial are typical. Longer term reactions include unpredictable emotions, flashbacks, strained relationships and even physical symptoms like headaches or nausea.
>
> (APA, 2022)

Centre for Addiction and Mental Health believes:

> Trauma is the lasting emotional response that often results from living through a distressing event. Experiencing a traumatic event can harm a person's sense of safety, sense of self, and ability to regulate emotions and navigate relationships. Long after the traumatic event occurs, people with trauma can often feel shame, helplessness, powerlessness and intense fear.
>
> (CAMH, 2022)

Trauma can be subdivided into primary and secondary categories. Primary trauma is the initial exposure with any major type of trauma that directly impacts the individual, whereas secondary or vicarious trauma denotes the indirect experience of witnessing or learning about another individual's trauma. Secondary trauma can be identified as "compassion fatigue, countertransference, and burnout" (Sweeney et al., 2018, p. 322). Therapists, healthcare practitioners, and service providers are at the receiving end of secondary trauma due to the empathic and close connections that occur within these dynamics; these interactions can potentially disrupt their healing journey.

Judith Herman (1992, 2022), a pioneering scholar in trauma-informed care, posits that there are three stages of recovery. The first stage is the establishment of safety (within our body, thoughts and emotions, and externally within our environment and connections), which is compromised after a traumatic event. This stage also incorporates stabilization and grounding. Stage two entails remembrance and mourning, during which the client and therapist co-construct and subsequently reauthor the trauma story; this simultaneously relinquishes guilt and shame about the traumatic event. The final stage, reconnection, encourages self-development, loving kindness, forgiveness, and taking care of oneself (i.e., mind, body, environment, interpersonal relationships, community) through deliberate and intentional activities. In my practice, I delineate between three types of behaviours that clients may demonstrate while moving through the stages of treatment: resistance, reluctance, and readiness. The readiness element represents a dichotomy between readiness and non-readiness. Therapy must introduce building coping skills to help clients reconcile ambivalence such that they sustain their readiness to heal.

Referencing the work of Francine Shapiro, founder of EMDR (eye movement desensitization and reprocessing therapy), trauma can take the form of Big T and little t. Big T consists of life-threatening events such as experiencing war, concentration camps, genocide, natural disasters, motor vehicle accidents, childhood abuse, domestic violence, diagnosis of a severe illness, or major surgeries. Little t traumas are also life-threatening but are more personal traumatic events; for example, racism, oppression, global crisis, divorce, bullying, emotional abuse, poverty, neglect, adoption, financial concerns, migrating to a new country, or workplace stress (Gilmoor et al., 2019; Shapiro, 2017).

Events

Adverse Childhood Experiences (ACEs) are traumatic events that can occur during one's childhood, prior to age 18. Due to monumental brain development, children between the ages of five and eight are theoretically at greater risk and the most vulnerable to trauma (Felitti et al., 2019; Perry & Winfrey, 2021). As part of my history taking with clients, I link how ACEs are relevant to their current core beliefs by means of exploring their truths, thoughts, emotions, and behaviours associated with these experiences. By discerning the overlap between the ACEs and client's present narrative, I enhance my understanding of the intricacies encapsulated in their past mindset. Ten ACEs are:

- Emotional abuse
- Physical abuse
- Sexual abuse
- Emotional neglect
- Physical neglect
- Household dysfunction/violence/divorced parents
- Mental illness
- "Loss" of a parent
- Incarcerated family member
- Substance (alcohol, drugs) use in home

Individuals who experience ACEs and have unresolved pediatric trauma from the past might encounter low mood/depression; health concerns such as heart disease, cancer, diabetes; suicidality; employment barriers; and substance use (Gilgoff et al., 2020). Some of these ACEs can be disputed via a cultural lens; they may not be completely accurate in terms of how BIPOC process Western perspectives regarding developmental or relational trauma. Events such as emotional or physical neglect might be represented differently or may be normalized within the culture. A BIPOC father who is processing his trauma may not be as talkative or as involved in his children's wellbeing, in which case the mother may overcompensate for this deficit. Listening to cultural nuances embedded within the client's narrative is essential to discern these disparities.

Additionally, traumatic events in the form of microaggressions, internalized racism, racial trauma, or intergenerational trauma can develop from or coexist with racism (Bombay et al., 2009; Comas-Díaz et al., 2019). To further clarify this matter, there are three Es that define trauma: event(s), experience of event(s), and effect(s) of the event (Lathan et al., 2021). Each factor builds on the previous factor. Table 1.1 is adapted from the Substance Abuse and Mental Health Services Administration (2014) definitions of the three Es:

Table 1.1 The three Es of trauma

Event	Experience	Effect
Trauma can either be real or a perceived threat.	Recognizing the variation of personalized responses/reactions to an event, specifically surrounding meaning-making and one's intersectionality.	Negative consequences can be delayed. Trauma can affect an individual's overall wellbeing and cognitive processes on either a short-term or long-term basis.
A single or a series of events over one's lifetime.	Power dynamics may ensue due to these events.	Daily coping and interpersonal relationships are impacted due to trauma, creating issues with trust.
Trauma can manifest in traditional forms such as abuse, violence, natural disasters, or via systemic oppression, namely racism, capitalism, or collective trauma such as the Holocaust, 1947 Partition of India/Pakistan, or the COVID-19 pandemic.	Emotions relevant to shame, guilt, and betrayal; lean into concerns with trust. Questioning event and feeling accountable to reinforce these emotions.	Effects related to trauma can include flashbacks, nightmares, dissociation, hypervigilance, paranoia, and perpetual arousal response. If trauma goes untreated, individuals may feel fatigued with ongoing symptoms.

Furthermore, it is essential to understand the four types of trauma: acute, chronic, complex, and system-induced. Acute trauma refers to an individual incident or single event (i.e., natural disaster, pandemic); chronic trauma occurs when the events are repetitious and prolonged (i.e., physical abuse, racism); complex trauma results from experiencing multiple, varied, and intrusive traumatic occurrences (i.e., a combination of a motor vehicle accident, domestic violence, abandonment); and the more recently coined system-induced trauma involves being exposed to previously helpful systems that become corrupt traumatic systems (i.e., educational system, foster care, sibling separation, immigration, healthcare system) (Bremner, 1999; Cummings et al., 2022). Treatment for these forms of trauma are EMDR and somatic experiencing, which both use brain-based and nervous system techniques to heal and move forward from trauma.

Effects

Effects of trauma can be recognized on both physical and psychological levels. For some, trauma can elicit somatic responses present as physical concerns such as headaches, disrupted sleep, lack of appetite, dizziness, headaches, and abdominal issues (Sodhi, 2017). On a psychological front, trauma can radiate to include symptoms associated with anxiety, depression, substance use, and post-traumatic stress disorder (PTSD). Trauma is multifaceted and is comprised of various contexts. Trauma is not exclusive to psychological constructs; one must understand how it impacts the nervous system and our overall biology. Trauma can sit in the body and appear in the form of serious physical health conditions (Maté, 2004; van der Kolk, 2014).

In session, when somatic sensations are detected in one's body, I ask clients, "Where are you feeling the discomfort?" "How would you articulate/name these sensations?" We mutually explore the pain and hurt that is stored in their bodies through a variety of systems and disciplines. Clients, society, and the profession of psychotherapy need to create a space to talk about trauma without feeling any shame. This can be achieved by destigmatizing trauma; using language that the person will understand; developing safety, trust, rapport, and relationship; and integrating these criteria into their existing ecosystems: home, academic setting, community, and host culture. This process of creating space needs to be tangential.

Trauma and the Brain

There has been tremendous and ground-breaking research about how trauma affects the mind and various parts of the brain, specifically the amygdala, hippocampus, and prefrontal cortex (Bremner, 2006; Perry &

Winfrey, 2021; Siegel, 1999; van der Kolk, 2014). Trauma can modify neural infrastructure and circuits, thus altering the nervous system and grey matter capacity (Sweeney et al., 2018). Many elements of treatment are underutilized with BIPOC, inclusive of the interplay between neuroscience (i.e., brain, polyvagal) and attachment and attunement; client perception and attachment to everyday figures and therapeutic alliance; using language to articulate trauma; positive history taking; brainspotting; and neurofeedback. EMDR is effectively used more in trauma-informed practices; however, most of these interventions require an amalgam of EMDR and cultural considerations (Ashley & Lipscomb, 2020; Nickerson, 2022).

EMDR can be facilitated in tandem with other therapeutic strategies such as mindfulness, psychoeducation, and select cognitive behavioural therapy (CBT) techniques such as understanding cognitive distortions and unhealthy beliefs (van den Hout et al., 2011). EMDR is an evidence-based psychotherapeutic treatment that attempts to mitigate symptoms associated with traumatic experiences, events, and memories (Shapiro, 1989). It is also known to treat PTSD, addictions, mood disorders, panic disorders, and phobias. This approach uses bilateral stimulation emerging from eye movement, taps, and tones, which assist in remembering rather than reliving trauma-related occurrences. Other benefits are processing trauma memories in a safe space, acquiring skills to expand upon distress tolerance, learning and applying mindfulness practices, and fostering positive self-beliefs. Clients are guided to process traumatic events which can decrease the intensity of the thoughts, feelings, and sensations associated with the experiences. EMDR consists of an eight-phase treatment plan: history taking session(s), client preparation, assessment, desensitization, installation, body scan, closure, and re-evaluation of treatment effect (Menon & Jayan, 2010).

There are multicultural implications that affect one's migratory trauma. Frequently what occurs in my work with clients is the need to share their narrative on a gradual basis by implementing the titration technique (which is covered in Chapter 3), a deliberate process that requires co-construction of the trauma narrative. This technique supports the client to define and name trauma so that it is not internalized. Often clients demonstrate some resistance towards engaging fully with disclosing their traumas; therapists assist the client ready themselves for contact with trauma wounds while walking alongside, validating their sentiments, and holding space for them.

Also remarkable is the positive impact of having a connected combination of Eastern and Western healers versus meeting with one Western trained health professional. I have observed resourceful clients in my own practice who have an interdisciplinary team or circle of care instead of meeting exclusively with their family doctor. Acccessing different perspectives allows clients more room for futher success and strategies to ameliorate and offer long-term results and overall positive wellbeing. It also suggests that loneliness, which may manifest as physical and mental health issues, may be precluded by social connectedness (Ikigai, a Japanese concept discussed in Chapter 7) (García & Miralles, 2017; Maté & Maté, 2022).

Core beliefs about guilt, shame, blame, and feeling culturally "never good enough" commonly surface in my conversations with BIPOC clients about trauma-related events. There is a stigma associated with naming and accepting the trauma that has shaped their present mindset. Brené Brown (2006) identifies four strategies to develop shame resilience:

1. Recognizing, naming, and understanding our shame triggers.
2. Identifying external factors that led to the feelings of shame.
3. Connecting with others to receive and offer empathy.
4. Speaking about our feelings of shame with others.

Each of these strategies foster inner growth and healing. Clients are motivated to seek connections with family and community, whom they deem safe. By voicing their thoughts and feelings about shame, clients develop a sense of idyllic empowerment and the ability to feel seen, heard, and supported. This inspires clients to let go of shame, build trust, and break intergenerational trauma cycles.

Chapter 2 outlines collective, cultural, and historical trauma. Trauma can be a result of cultural legacy burdens (systemic oppression from the host culture), family legacy burdens (from immediate or extended family), and individual legacy burdens (microaggressions) (Gutiérrez, 2022; Schwartz, 2021). One's core beliefs, values, and needs may also inform how intergenerational trauma might manifest differently from culture to culture.

The next chapter offers information about myths and relevant types of trauma, as well as a table outlining the latter.

References

American Psychiatric Association, DSM-5 Task Force. (2013). *Diagnostic and statistical manual of mental disorders: DSM-5* (5th ed.). American Psychiatric Publishing, Inc.

American Psychological Association (APA). (2022). *Trauma*. Retrieved March 1, 2022, from www.apa.org/topics/trauma

Ashley, W., & Lipscomb, A. (2020). Addressing racialized trauma, utilizing EMDR and antiracist psychotherapy practices. *EMDR and Racial Trauma. EMDR and Racial Trauma Special Edition in Go with That Magazine, EMDRIA.Org, 25*(3), 22–26.

Bombay, A., Matheson, K., & Anisman, H. (2009). Intergenerational trauma: Convergence of multiple processes among First Nations peoples in Canada. *International Journal of Indigenous Health*, 5(3), 6–47.

Bremner, J. D. (1999). Acute and chronic responses to psychological trauma: Where do we go from here? *The American Journal of Psychiatry*, 156(3), 349–351.

Bremner, J. D. (2006). Traumatic stress: Effects on the brain. *Dialogues in Clinical Neuroscience*, 8(4), 445–461.

Brown, B. (2006). Shame resilience theory: A grounded theory study on women and shame. *Families in Society*, 87(1), 43–52.

Centre for Addiction and Mental Health (CAMH). (2022). Retrieved October 8, 2022, from www.camh.ca/en/health-info/mental-illness-and-addiction-index/trauma

Comas-Díaz, L., Hall, G. N., & Neville, H. A. (2019). Racial trauma: Theory, research, and healing: Introduction to the special issue. *American Psychologist*, 74(1), 1–5.

Cummings, A. D. P., Clark, T. J., Conrad, C. G., & Johnson, A. D. (2022) Trauma: Community of color exposure to the criminal justice system as an adverse childhood experience. *University of Cincinnati Law Review*, 90(3), 857–922.

Felitti, V. J., Anda, R. F., Nordenberg, D., Williamson, D. F., Spitz, A. M., Edwards, V., & Marks, J. S. (2019). Relationship of childhood abuse and household dysfunction to many of the leading causes of death in adults: The adverse childhood experiences (ACE) study. *American Journal of Preventive Medicine*, 56(6), 774–786.

García, H., & Miralles, F. (2017). *IKIGAI: The Japanese secret to living a long and happy life*. Penguin Life.

Gilgoff, R., Singh, L., Koita, K., Gentile, B., & Marques, S. S. (2020). Adverse childhood experiences, outcomes, and interventions. *Pediatric Clinics of North America*, 67(2), 259–273.

Gilmoor, A. R., Adithy, A., & Regeer, B. (2019). The cross-cultural validity of post-traumatic stress disorder and post-traumatic stress symptoms in the Indian context: A systematic search and review. *Frontiers in Psychiatry*, 10, 439, 1–24.

Gutiérrez, N. Y. (2022). *The pain we carry: Healing from complex PTSD for people of color*. New Harbinger Publications Inc.

Herman, J. L. (1992). *Trauma and recovery*. Basic Books.

Herman, J. L. (2022). *Trauma and recovery: The aftermath of violence – From domestic abuse to political terror*. Basic Books.

Lathan, E. C., Selwyn, C. N., & Langhinrichsen-Rohling, J. (2021). The "3 Es" of trauma-informed care in a federally qualified health center: Traumatic event and experience-related predictors of physical and mental health effects among female patients. *Journal of Community Psychology*, 49(2), 703–724.

Maté, G. (2004). *When the body says no: The cost of hidden stress*. Vintage Canada.

Maté, G., & Maté, D. (2022). *The myth of normal: Trauma, illness, and healing in a toxic culture*. Avery.

Menon, S. B., & Jayan, C. (2010). Eye movement desensitization and reprocessing: A conceptual framework. *Indian Journal of Psychological Medicine*, 32(2), 136–140.

Nickerson, M. (Ed.). (2022). *Cultural competence and healing culturally based trauma with EMDR therapy: Innovative strategies and protocols*. Springer Publishing Company.

Perry, B., & Winfrey, O. (2021). *What happened to you?* Flatiron Books.

Schwartz, R. C. (2021). *No bad parts: Healing trauma and restoring wholeness with the internal family systems model.* Sounds True.

Shapiro, F. (1989). Efficacy of the eye movement desensitization procedure in the treatment of traumatic memories. *Journal of Traumatic Stress, 2*(2), 199–223.

Shapiro, F. (2017). *Eye movement desensitization and reprocessing (EMDR) therapy: Basic principles, protocols and procedures* (3rd ed.). Guilford Press.

Siegel, D. J. (1999). *The developing mind: How relationships and the brain interact to shape who we are.* Guilford Press.

Sodhi, P. K. (2017). *Exploring immigrant and sexual minority mental health: Reconsidering multiculturalism.* Routledge.

Substance Abuse and Mental Health Services Administration (SAMHSA). (2014). *SAMHSA's concept of trauma and guidance for a trauma-informed approach (HHS Publication No. SMA 14–4884).* Substance Abuse and Mental Health Services Administration.

Sweeney, A., Filson, B., Kennedy, A., Collinson, L., & Gillard, S. (2018). A paradigm shift: Relationships in trauma-informed mental health services. *BJPsych Advances, 24*(5), 319–333.

van den Hout, M. A., Engelhard, I. M., Beetsma, D., Slofstra, C., Hornsveld, H., Houtveen, J., & Leer, A. (2011). EMDR and mindfulness. Eye movements and attentional breathing tax working memory and reduce vividness and emotionality of aversive ideation. *Journal of Behavior Therapy and Experimental Psychiatry, 42*(4), 423–431.

van der Kolk, B. (2014). *The body keeps the score: Mind, brain and body in the transformation of trauma.* Penguin Books.

Chapter 2

Myths and Types of Trauma

For BIPOC, trauma discourses expand beyond PTSD and intergenerational migratory hardships. This chapter provides an overview of myths and types of trauma experienced by BIPOC and the associated impact these traumas continue to have on their mental health.

Myths

One of the implicit intentions of this book is to discredit myths about trauma experienced by BIPOC clients. There are a variety of inquiries and myths that continue to garner ample attention. Common inquiries include the following:

Does epigenetic trauma exist?
What constitutes a cycle breaker?
How does one become retraumatized?
What differentiates individual from community healing?
At what age is one most vulnerable to the effects of trauma?
How accessible and culturally responsive is the *DSM-5* towards BIPOC?

Here are some myths:

Trauma healing involves forgiveness.
One can never heal from traumatic pain.
Trauma victims can never feel safe again.
Ignoring the trauma will make it go away.
Time and patience help heal trauma-related wounds.
Therapy does not help with trauma-related presenting concerns.
Only war survivors can experience post-traumatic stress disorder (PTSD).

Throughout this chapter and remainder of the book, I challenge and decolonize these myths and present better knowledge about trauma and how it affects BIPOC.

DOI: 10.4324/9781003216568-4

Types of Trauma

The following is a non-exhaustive list outlining a range of traumas experienced by BIPOC individuals:

- Colonial trauma
- Cultural trauma
- Developmental trauma
- Intersectional trauma
- Post-traumatic stress disorder (PTSD)/Complex post-traumatic stress disorder (C-PTSD)
- Migratory trauma
- Systemic trauma
- Collective trauma

In this text, more attention is given to racial and intergenerational trauma as they significantly pertain to BIPOC communities.

Colonial Trauma

Due to its ability to immobilize and denigrate BIPOC communities, colonial trauma can result in *collective* psychological and emotional harm; both can be intergenerational and span throughout one's lifetime (Mitchell & Maracle, 2005). It can originate from past genocidal events, which may produce suffering on a psychological and medical front. Often related to the global colonization of the Indigenous populations, colonial trauma directly impacts individuals on mental and physical health levels (Mitchell et al., 2019). Within North America, an example of colonial trauma entails the displacement of Indigenous peoples from their land and the imposed residential schools, all of which compromised Indigenous peoples' cultural identity, sense of belonging, and spiritual way of being (Nelson & Wilson, 2017). These topics are further analyzed in Part 2 of this book.

Cultural Trauma

Alexander (2016) suggests, "cultural trauma occurs when members of a collective feel they have been subjected to a horrendous event that leaves indelible marks upon their group consciousness, marking their memories forever and changing their future identity in fundamental and irrevocable ways" (p. 1). August 15, 2022, commemorated the 75th anniversary of India's freedom and independence from the British rule. For most Indian immigrants, it was a time to pay homage and reflect on our ancestral culture's narrative, yet for my family, it holds an assortment of emotions, nostalgia, and cultural trauma:

> *Over the years, my parents shared milder iterations of their "Partition stories." As I became older, I asked them to elaborate further on their*

experiences. My mother's childhood narrative involved her parents and six sisters, living in "Pakistan" at the time. My grandfather decided to shift his medical practice to "India" in June of 1947. With the help of his Muslim friends, the entire family boarded a train and safely arrived in "India." My mother said if they had postponed their trip by even one week, they would have never reached "India." She referenced "blood" and "ghost" trains that never made it to their destinations.

Relatedly, as mentioned in the introduction, during the turbulent 1980s, our family of five travelled to Punjab, India. We experienced strict curfews, required "special" visas to enter Punjab, were followed by police throughout the Golden Temple (the holiest Sikh shrine in India), and heard about several close-by bus bombings. My parents deliberately scheduled our departure flights to Canada after August 15th in case another bombing happened on this national holiday. Upon our return to Canada, we processed our trauma, grief, and anxiety together.

I was unable to name these events cultural trauma until recently; I now understand why these topics were silenced rather than discussed when we travelled abroad to see extended family.

Developmental Trauma

Dr. Gabor Maté talks extensively about developmental trauma (also known as relational trauma) and the influence it has on infants, children, and adolescents (Maté & Maté, 2022). Such trauma could involve repeated exposure and creations of abandonment, neglect, and betrayal wounds, different types of abuse, assault (e.g., emotional, physical, or sexual), or witnessing violence or deaths within the familial dynamic. Trauma that occurs during one's gestation and childhood can affect brain development and possibly result in long-term trauma-related symptoms and/or psychiatric conditions (van de Kolk, 2005).

Utero trauma is commonly caused by chaotic or unpredictable lifestyle factors including, but not limited to, the mother's exposure to domestic violence, familial discord, lack of antenatal care, or substance misuse during pregnancy (Lehner & Yehuda, 2018). Stress experienced by the mother can lead to increased levels of cortisol (stress hormone) in her body, which can then be passed onto her unborn child via the placenta. Elevated levels of cortisol and foetal distress can impact brain development and possibly change unique architectural and organizational features (Perry & Winfrey, 2021). This can result in reduced and impaired physical and mental functioning, which can devolve into lifelong implications for the child such as low birth weight and head circumference; neurobehavioural abnormalities; impairment of normal brain development and functioning (learning capacity, emotional regulation and stability, attachment issues, physical co-ordination, and/or self-esteem); anxiety and depression; and the inability to form healthy attachments with others (Reynolds et al., 2013).

Similarly, adverse childhood experiences (as noted in Chapter 1) support the notion that this type of trauma shapes one's adult mindset. Repercussions of developmental trauma can appear during one's adulthood in one's interpersonal relationships, dynamics with one's children, or interactions with other family members.

Intersectional Trauma

Not as commonly discussed, intersectional trauma recognizes how diverse aspects of one's identity respond to stress or "invisible trauma" (Sweeney et al., 2018). It explores how oppressive systems (e.g., colonialism, racism, sexism, homophobia) and community, cultural, and social contexts affects one's intersectionality (e.g., race, culture, gender, sexual orientation, ability, social class) (Crenshaw, 1991). Depending on how one is socialized or raised, intersectional trauma can manifest in how one accesses help and how one processes both guilt and shame. Intersectional trauma can yield a variety of internalized and unresolved stress/trauma responses.

Post-Traumatic Stress Disorder (Ptsd)/Complex Post-Traumatic Stress Disorder (C-Ptsd)

Post-traumatic stress disorder (PTSD) is "a natural reaction to a deeply shocking and disturbing experience. It is a normal reaction to an abnormal situation" which lasts over one month (American Psychiatric Association, 2013). Often what transpires is the reliving of traumatic events via insomnia, lack of concentration, depression, anger, stress, nightmares, anxiety flashbacks, low self-esteem, and panic attacks. For BIPOC, PTSD and depression are common for those who experience familial, ancestral, and identity-related losses (Sodhi, 2017). Other factors, such as physical and sexual abuse, witnessing violent acts, displacement from their ancestral country by war, and residing in refugee camps could contribute to post-traumatic stress related symptoms in children and intensify pre-existing PTSD symptoms in adults and children alike (Guo et al., 2023; Kirmayer et al., 2011). Complex post-traumatic stress disorder (C-PTSD) arises from a combination of chronic or repeated traumatic events at any stage of an individual's life. van der Kolk (2014) states that C-PTSD can produce disruption with memory and attention, maladaptive coping strategies, low self-perception, issues with regulation of affect and impulses, toxic interpersonal relationships, and somatization of trauma stored in the body.

Migratory Trauma

Initiated by trauma experienced in the country of origin, mental health issues may surface upon migrating to another country. These concerns could include depression/anxiety related to the immigration and resettlement process, depression attributed to isolation/poverty, depression/anxiety due to loss of identity, and adjustment disorder (Sodhi, 2017). Premigration narratives are imperative in conceptualizing immigrant mental health. Life-threatening events (e.g., war and genocide), economic insecurities, physical and sexual abuse, and death of or separation from family members have been closely linked to mood disorders, borderline personality disorder, schizophrenia, and C-PTSD within immigrant populations. Unfortunately, coming to terms with these mental health conditions may have an effect on an immigrant's adjustment within the host country. Compounding these potential diagnoses, sources of ambivalence or internal conflict such as motives to migrate, reasons to stay, and barriers to leave may create unrealistic visions and expectations of the ancestral country and uncertainty of immigrating to a new country.

Systemic Trauma

Systemic trauma denotes the trauma that might occur within physical environments such as educational institutions, religious venues, workplace milieus, penitentiaries, and healthcare settings. It can encompass migratory or immigration challenges, racism and discrimination, sexism, homophobia, police brutality, microaggressions, racial profiling, community violence, and dated laws. I elaborate on all of the aforementioned settings, as well as how these types of trauma are created and then dismantled within our society (Goldsmith et al., 2014; Khasnabis & Goldin, 2020; Kira et al., 2014).

Collective Trauma

"Collective trauma refers to the psychological reactions to a traumatic event that affect an entire society; it does not merely reflect a historical fact or the recollection of a terrible event that happened to a group of people" (Hirschberger, 2018, p. 1). Collective trauma that affects future generations is called intergenerational trauma. Implications of collective trauma that are commonly discussed by BIPOC are mentioned here:

- Feeling disconnected from the world.
- Encountering unusual forms of overt and covert racism.
- Fearing the unknown/future leading to catastrophic thinking.
- Grieving life before the traumatic event and living in the past.

- Reduced capacity to cope with chronic anxiety, depression, and stress.
- Loss of interest in daily activities and socializing with others.
- Existential dread and reconsidering one's meaning and purpose in life.

Collective trauma can affect a community, town, village, country, or become a global event where one might feel immense change and loss. Examples of these events include the Holocaust, World Wars, 9/11, and the COVID-19 pandemic.

Racial Trauma

Racial trauma (also known as race-based traumatic stress) refers to the stressors and physical/emotional wounds that an individual incurs due to cumulative exposure to racism and discrimination (Comas-Díaz et al., 2019). Dr. Kenneth Hardy (2013, 2023) succinctly identifies the hidden wounds of racial trauma: internalized devaluation, assaulted sense of self, internalized voicelessness, and the wound of rage. Describing each of these injuries as such supports the targeted individual to understand how racial trauma activates different parts of their being. Taking space to attend to these wounds and redirecting feelings of anger, rage, and helplessness is imperative to the healing process.

Over the last two decades, several shootings, targeted killings, and premeditated hate crimes have transpired post-9/11. BIPOC continue to feel oppressed, attacked, and targeted by colonial capitalist white supremacist acts of violence, police brutality, and gun culture. The impact is real, and the repercussions of these traumatic events reverberate within their nervous systems and compromise their mental health (Williams et al., 2022).

Mental health implications from racial trauma are as follows:

- Anxiety
- Depression
- Chronic stress
- Somatization of emotional pain
- Substance use disorders
- Post-traumatic stress disorder (PTSD)

Symptoms of these mental health conditions can manifest in assorted ways:

- Relationship challenges
- Fear for personal safety
- Distrust and withdrawing from the world

- Disrupted sleep, insomnia, and nightmares
- Intrusive/recurring thoughts or images
- Heightened sensitivity to threat and shaming
- Arousal in the form of hypervigilance and increased suspicion
- Negative cognitions about self, society, and the world
- Increased aggression and potential domestic violence

Correspondingly, discrepancies exist between white and racialized media coverage, such as BIPOC representation. In short, members of marginalized communities are not receiving the same news coverage or acknowledgement of community tragedy as are white individuals. This variation is apparent insofar as current day BIPOC hate crimes receive less attention than do cases of "missing white women syndrome." By amplifying news concerning white individuals, we are undermining the lives of racialized and ethnic individuals and prolonging the colonial belief of not mattering.

Intergenerational Trauma

Intergenerational trauma (also known as transgenerational trauma and ancestral trauma) alludes to the phenomenon of a traumatic event experienced by a previous generation impacting the current generation. This process starts with a traumatic event which may affect an individual, a family, a community, or cultural/ethnic/racial groups; in the case of the latter two scenarios, such trauma could also be said to be collective. Historical trauma is a subtype or derivation of intergenerational trauma. It may be comprised of intergenerational transmission of wounds, trauma responses, psychological manifestations, and healing and coping strategies (Fisher, 2017). It can arise via parenting, cultural practices, systemic policies and structures, and personalized traumas.

Intergenerational trauma can result from racial trauma or other systemic oppression (e.g., colonialism), examples of which include but are not limited to, the Holocaust, the 1947 Partition of India/Pakistan, enslavement, and the residential school system. Intergenerational trauma can be internalized in a multitude of ways: physical and emotional abuse, substance use disorders, autoimmune disease, undiagnosed mental health conditions, heightened anxiety, depression, suicidality, mistrust, fear of the future, codependency, panic attacks, insomnia, dissociations, inability to establish trust, lack of security or safety, low self-confidence, shame and guilt, intrusive thoughts, emotional numbness and dysregulation, people pleasing tendencies, and lack of identity or belonging (Sodhi, 2023).

If intergenerational trauma is left unresolved or unhealed, it can permeate into social, psychological, and epigenetic aspects of one's being (Gameon & Skewes, 2020). Genes relevant to epigenetic trauma are passed down and leave biomarkers on one's DNA. This epigenetic alteration might alter one's life choices and mental health (Lehrner & Yehuda, 2018). Breaking an intergenerational cycle challenges the expression of these biomarkers so that they are not further transmitted to future generations (Maté & Maté, 2022; Williams et al., 2022). Epigenetic modifications within the brain can be reversed through somatic experiencing, hypnosis, mindfulness-based stress reduction (MBSR) techniques (e.g., meditation), neuro-linguistic programming (NLP), medications, neurofeedback, cognitive behavioural therapy (CBT), eye movement desensitization and reprocessing (EMDR), and other brain-related modalities (Cao-Lei et al., 2022; Yehuda et al., 2013).

As trauma is inherently an injury to relationships, it behooves us to consider not only the types of trauma but the roles that different individuals may play in the disruption or maintenance of it. Such an examination follows.

Individual Roles

Cycle Breakers

Cycle breakers are often villainized within family systems regarding their efforts to disrupt epigenetics and unlearn unhealthy/toxic patterns that transcend from previous generations (Islam et al., 2022; St. Laurent et al., 2019). These individuals deviate from the family collective due to their recognition of perilous coping strategies. Instead, they choose not to repeat history, replace these practices by initiating the familial healing process, and therefore gain a better understanding of their family's potential actions and behaviours. These changes take place while the individual is learning more about their intersectionality outside of their familial dynamic. Similarly, neuroplasticity could assist in changing the cerebral hardwiring of the brain by unlearning and relearning (Doidge, 2015; Winship, 2019). Comparable to immigrants who assimilate within a new culture, some individuals may encounter a grieving process necessary for change to take place (Sodhi, 2017; Wexler, 2006, 2010). Grief (as a cycle breaker) in this context might look like letting go of people pleasing tendencies with a more empowered and boundaried disposition.

Cycle Maintainers

Contrary to cycle breakers, "cycle maintainers" are individuals who perpetuate and normalize intergenerational trauma (St. Laurent et al., 2019). Naming and processing traumatic events prevalent within our ancestral narratives can forestall future lineage from becoming cycle maintainers;

this practice is not only for the present generation, but for one's ancestors and future generations – it is a collective effort. By doing so, we are not only healing individual pain but also familial pain, ancestor pain, and community pain. Cycle breakers need to share and discuss the good and bad moments of their ancestral narrative so future lineage are not obliged to break the cycle for the previous generation.

If trauma can transcend generations, so can healing by breaking or *smashing* intergenerational cycles. This happens visually and auditorily by amplifying one's voice. Healing intergenerational trauma and sacred wounds occurs on emotional, mental, physical, and somatic levels. As trauma is transmitted from generation to generation, it is necessary to recognize and learn about the root cause of what is ultimately being activated within one's nervous system. Intergenerational cycles can be broken; however, processing, unlearning, and healing must occur between these cycles.

Reclamation Process

The reclamation process encourages cycle breakers to name and reclaim the origins of their ancestor's trauma, externalize what has been passed down (e.g., shame, guilt, cultural/familial/individual legacy burdens), and participate in relevant healing practices. It involves engaging in deep introspective and intentional ancestral work to remove the mark that has been transmitted and avoid the internalization of one's parents' trauma narratives. Even though cycle breakers are healing within cycles that continue to repeat amidst the cycle maintainers around them, other events may start to stagnate their healing process and build upon existing layers of intergenerational trauma. The reclamation process warrants unpacking, understanding, and relinquishing all trauma-related symptoms.

Over the years, select family members may have exhibited "generational tolerance"; some of these family members may demonstrate their own progression. As individuals, they may have shifted from complacency to feeling conflicted to becoming more assertive and standing up for their own rights. Cycle breakers emerge when they are ready to look within, detach, and do the necessary therapeutic work to heal their traumatic ancestral wounds. By attending therapy, individuals nurture their mental health and can learn strategies to deconstruct, break intergenerational trauma cycles, and acquire intergenerational resilience (Denov et al., 2019; Isobel et al., 2021; Kazlauskas et al., 2017). Having one's trauma narrative heard and understood in a safe and validating space contributes to the healing process.

Healing From Trauma

An individual can start the healing process by using a genogram to help clarify intergenerational trauma and relationships, roles, life experiences, migratory concerns, and family history; unpack cultural and historical layers ingrained within trauma-related symptoms; develop a secure and positive self-identity; improve upon their (present/future) parenting style by not transmitting displaced or emotional distress to offspring; replace unhealthy familial dialogue with affirmative communication (Sells, 2018); rewrite intergenerational trauma narratives with the intention of breaking the cycle; and abstain from becoming activated or responding to similar trauma in a similar manner as did their ancestors.

Alternatively, initiating factual discussions and identifying traumatic events with family (e.g., grandparents, parents, aunts, uncles, siblings, children) is fundamental to breaking cycles of intergenerational trauma. What does this entail?

- Keeping lines of communication open regarding trauma. Recognize overt and covert emotions, responses, and reactions to current traumatic news. Reassure physical and emotional safety.
- Acknowledging the link between the history of systemic oppression and current global events. Make every event a learning opportunity.
- Overcoming collective grief can include becoming a productive ally to BIPOC who have dealt with diverse forms of trauma. Experiential activism encourages intergenerational families to participate in writing letters, signing petitions, attending vigils, and posting factual information on social media platforms. Exemplifying these actions through various mediums will influence future generations to consistently stand together to eradicate racial injustice. Ultimately, intergenerational communication strengthens intergenerational resilience and fosters curiosity to learn more about these timely topics.

Example of Intergenerational Trauma

Figure 2.1 illustrates an example of intergenerational trauma. World events such as enslavement, the Holocaust, and the 1947 Partition of India/Pakistan stoke a variety of trauma-related responses. The effects of these events continue to modify my BIPOC clients' daily existences, perceptions of the world, and interactions with others. This type of trauma continues to affect populations for generations after a collective traumatic event has occurred and can cause widespread nervous system dysregulation. For example, if enslavement led to severe mental health conditions and substance use disorders in a client's grandparents, the client may have been affected by this through their parents' mood fluctuations, depression, people pleasing tendencies, anxiety, or codependency. As cycle breakers, my clients learn more about the traits associated with carrying ancestral trauma, explore unresolved guilt and shame, confront and overcome their culturally specific inner child wounds (i.e., abandonment, neglect, guilt, and trust concerns), develop inner resiliency, and eventually become more resilient by applying the inclusion and healing therapy (IHT) framework introduced in Part 4 of this book.

As mentioned in Figure 2.1, the concepts of indirect and direct intergenerational trauma deserve attention. Trauma can be passed down from generation to generation; it can also skip a generation (e.g., grandparents to grandchildren). Skipping generations could be a result of individual efforts to break cycles; heal between cycles; and/or a product of what the current generation was exposed to from previous relatives/ancestors. A reflective account of the client's ancestral narrative or their need to have the power

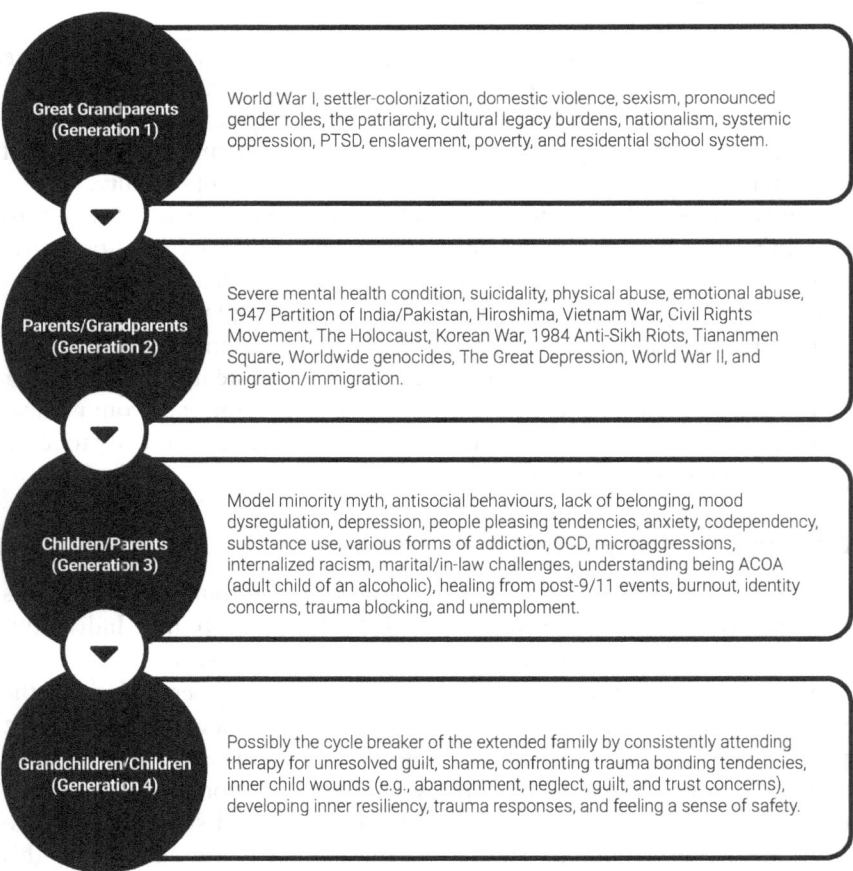

Figure 2.1 Four generations of trauma

and control over the trauma cycle would likely illustrate how trauma was indirectly transmitted to them.

To conclude, Table 2.1 offers a summary of the different kinds of trauma noted in this chapter.

Table 2.1 Types of trauma

Type of Trauma	Definition
Colonial Trauma	Resulting from collective psychological and emotional harm; it can be intergenerational, and can span throughout one's lifetime (Mitchell & Maracle, 2005). For example medical and psychological suffering produced by genocide.
Cultural Trauma	"When members of a collective culture feel they have been subjected to a horrendous event that leaves indelible marks upon their group consciousness, marking their memories forever and changing their future identity in fundamental and irrevocable ways" (Alexander, 2016).
Developmental Trauma	Exposure to repeated events or situations involving creations of abandonment, neglect, betrayal wounds, different types of abuse, assault (e.g., emotional, physical, or sexual), witnessing violence, or deaths within the familial dynamic.
Intersectional Trauma	How diverse aspects of one's identity respond to stress or "invisible trauma" (Sweeney et al., 2018). Refers to how oppressive systems (e.g., colonialism, racism, sexism, homophobia), community, and cultural and social contexts influence one's intersectionality (e.g., race, culture, gender, sexual orientation, ability, social class) (Crenshaw, 1991).
Post-Traumatic Stress Disorder (PTSD)/ Complex Post-Traumatic Stress Disorder (C-PTSD)	Post-traumatic stress disorder (PTSD) is "a natural reaction to a deeply shocking and disturbing experience. It is a normal reaction to an abnormal situation" which lasts over one month (American Psychiatric Association, 2013). Complex post-traumatic stress disorder (C-PTSD) originates from a combination of chronic or repeated traumatic events at any stage of an individual's life.
Migratory Trauma	Initiated by trauma experienced in the country of origin, mental health issues may surface upon migrating to another country. These concerns could include depression/anxiety related to the immigration and resettlement process, depression attributed to isolation/poverty, depression/anxiety due to loss of identity, and adjustment disorder (Sodhi, 2017).

(Continued)

Table 2.1 (Continued)

Type of Trauma	Definition
Systemic Trauma	Refers to the trauma that might occur within physical environments such as educational institutions, religious venues, workplace milieus, penitentiaries, and healthcare settings. It can involve migratory or immigration challenges, racism and discrimination, sexism, homophobia, police brutality, microaggressions, racial profiling, community violence, and dated laws.
Collective Trauma	"The psychological reactions to a traumatic event that affect an entire society; it does not merely reflect a historical fact or the recollection of a terrible event that happened to a group of people" (Hirschberger, 2018, p. 1). Collective trauma that affects future generations is called intergenerational trauma.
Racial Trauma	Racial trauma (also known as race-based traumatic stress) refers to the stressors and physical/emotional wounds that an individual experiences because of cumulative exposure to racism and discrimination (Comas-Díaz et al., 2019).
Intergenerational Trauma	Intergenerational trauma encompasses a previously experienced traumatic event that impacts the current generation. Historical trauma is a subtype or derivation of intergenerational trauma. It may be comprised of intergenerational transmission of wounds, trauma responses, psychological manifestations, and healing and coping strategies, and may skip generations.

The next chapter offers a compilation of culturally responsive trauma-informed practices. The relevancy of these approaches are applied to the narratives in Part 3 and within the inclusion and healing therapy (IHT) framework in Chapter 9.

References

Alexander, J. C. (2016). Culture trauma, morality and solidarity: The social construction of "Holocaust" and other mass murders. *Thesis Eleven, 132*, 3–16.

American Psychiatric Association, DSM-5 Task Force. (2013). *Diagnostic and statistical manual of mental disorders: DSM-5* (5th ed.). American Psychiatric Publishing, Inc.

Cao-Lei, L., Saumier, D., Fortin, J., & Brunet, A. (2022). A narrative review of the epigenetics of post-traumatic stress disorder and post-traumatic stress disorder treatment. *Frontiers in Psychiatry, 13*, 857087.

Comas-Díaz, L., Hall, G. N., & Neville, H. A. (2019). Racial trauma: Theory, research, and healing: Introduction to the special issue. *American Psychologist, 74*(1), 1–5.

Crenshaw, K. (1991). Mapping the margins: Intersectionality, identity politics, and violence against women of color. *Stanford Law Review, 43*(6), 1241–1299.

Denov, M., Fennig, M., Rabiau, M. A., & Shevell, M. C. (2019). Intergenerational resilience in families affected by war, displacement, and migration: "It runs in the family". *Journal of Family Social Work, 22*(1), 17–45.

Doidge, N. (2015). *The brain's way of healing: Remarkable discoveries and recoveries from the frontiers of neuroplasticity*. Penguin Books.

Fisher, J. (2017). *Healing the fragmented selves of trauma survivors: Overcoming internal self-alienation*. Routledge.

Gameon, J. A., & Skewes, M. C. (2020). A systematic review of trauma interventions in Native communities. *American Journal of Community Psychology, 65*(1–2), 223–241.

Goldsmith, R. E., Martin, C. G., & Smith, C. P. (2014). Systemic trauma. *Journal of Trauma & Dissociation: The Official Journal of the International Society for the Study of Dissociation (ISSD), 15*(2), 117–132.

Guo, L., Li, L., Xu, K., Wang, W., Ni, Y., Li, W., Gong, J., Lu, C., & Zhang, W. H. (2023). Characterization of premigration and postmigration multidomain factors and psychosocial health among refugee children and adolescents after resettlement in Australia. *JAMA Network Open, 6*(4), e235841.

Hardy, K. V. (2013). Healing the hidden wounds of racial trauma. *Reclaiming Children and Youth, 22*(1), 24–28.

Hardy, K. V. (2023). *Racial trauma: Clinical strategies and techniques for healing invisible wounds*. Norton Professional Books.

Hirschberger, G. (2018). Collective trauma and the social construction of meaning. *Frontiers in Psychology, 9*, 1441, 1–14.

Islam, S., Jaffee, S. R., & Widom, C. S. (2022). Breaking the cycle of intergenerational childhood maltreatment: Effects on offspring mental health. *Child Maltreatment, 28*(1), 119–129, 1–11.

Isobel, S., McCloughen, A., Goodyear, M., & Foster, K. (2021). Intergenerational trauma and its relationship to mental healthcare: A qualitative inquiry. *Community Mental Health Journal, 57*(4), 631–643.

Kazlauskas, E., Gailiene, D., Vaskeliene, I., & Skeryte-Kazlauskiene, M. (2017). Intergenerational transmission of resilience? Sense of coherence is associated between Lithuanian survivors of political violence and their adult offspring. *Frontiers in Psychology, 8*(1677), 1–8.

Khasnabis, D., & Goldin, S. (2020). Don't be fooled, trauma is a systemic problem: Trauma as a case of weaponized educational innovation. *Occasional Paper Series, 2020*(43), 44–58.

Kira, I., Lewandowski, L., Chiodo, L., & Ibrahim, A. (2014). Advances in systemic trauma theory: Traumatogenic dynamics and consequences of backlash as a multi-systemic trauma on Iraqi refugee Muslim adolescents. *Psychology, 5*, 389–412.

Kirmayer, L. J., Narasiah, L., Munoz, M., Rashid, M., Ryder, A. G., Guzder, J., Hassan, G., Rousseau, C., Pottie, K., & Canadian Collaboration for Immigrant and Refugee Health (CCIRH). (2011). Common mental health problems in immigrants and refugees: General approach in primary care. *CMAJ: Canadian Medical Association Journal, 183*(12), E959–E967.

Lehrner, A., & Yehuda, R. (2018). Cultural trauma and epigenetic inheritance. *Development and Psychopathology, 30*(5), 1763–1777.

Maté, G., & Maté, D. (2022). *The myth of normal: Trauma, illness, and healing in a toxic culture*. Knopf Canada.

Mitchell, T. L., Arseneau, C., & Thomas, D. (2019). Colonial trauma: Complex, continuous, collective, cumulative and compounding effects on the health of Indigenous peoples in Canada and beyond. *International Journal of Indigenous Health, 14*(2), 74–94.

Mitchell, T. L., & Maracle, D. T. (2005). Post-traumatic stress and the health status of Aboriginal populations in Canada. *Journal of Aboriginal Health, 2*(1), 14–23.

Nelson, S. E., & Wilson, K. (2017). The mental health of Indigenous peoples in Canada: A critical review of research. *Social Science and Medicine, 176*, 93–112.

Perry, B., & Winfrey, O. (2021). *What happened to you?* Flatiron Books.

Reynolds, R. M., Labad, J., Buss, C., Ghaemmaghami, P., & Räikkönen, K. (2013). Transmitting biological effects of stress in utero: Implications for mother and offspring. *Psychoneuroendocrinology, 38*(9), 1843–1849.

Sells, S. (2018). *A family systems approach to treating intergenerational trauma*. Retrieved February 21, 2021, from https://familytrauma.com/a-family-systems-approach-to-treating-intergenerational-trauma/

Sodhi, P. K. (2017). *Exploring immigrant and sexual minority mental health: Reconsidering multiculturalism*. Routledge.

Sodhi, P. K. (2023). Trauma-informed approaches for current and future lawyers. Webinar presented to the *Women's Legal Mentorship Program*, Ottawa, Ontario, January 26, 2023.

St-Laurent, D., Dubois-Comtois, K., Milot, T., & Cantinotti, M. (2019). Intergenerational continuity/discontinuity of child maltreatment among low-income mother-child dyads: The roles of childhood maltreatment characteristics, maternal psychological functioning, and family ecology. *Development and Psychopathology, 31*(1), 189–202.

Sweeney, A., Filson, B., Kennedy, A., Collinson, L., & Gillard, S. (2018). A paradigm shift: Relationships in trauma-informed mental health services. *BJPsych Advances, 24*(5), 319–333.

van der Kolk, B. A. (2005). Developmental trauma disorder: Toward a rational diagnosis for children with complex trauma histories. *Psychiatric Annals, 35*, 401–408.

van der Kolk, B. A. (2014). *The body keeps the score: Mind, brain and body in the transformation of trauma*. Penguin Books.

Wexler, B. E. (2006). *Brain and culture: Neurobiology, ideology and social change*. MIT Press.

Wexler, B. E. (2010). Neuroplasticity, cultural evolution and cultural difference. *World Cultural Psychiatry Research Review*, 11–22.

Williams, M. T., Khanna, R. A., & MacIntyre, M. P. (2022). The traumatizing impact of racism in Canadians of colour. *Current Trauma Reports, 8*(2), 17–34.

Winship, A. (2019). *Neuroplasticity: Exercises to improve cognitive flexibility, conquer trauma & PTSD, change bad habits, eliminate depression and so much more!* Josiah Vergonio.

Yehuda, R., Daskalakis, N. P., Desarnaud, F., Makotkine, I., Lehrner, A. L., Koch, E., Flory, J. D., Buxbaum, J. D., Meaney, M. J., & Bierer, L. M. (2013). Epigenetic biomarkers as predictors and correlates of symptom improvement following psychotherapy in combat veterans with PTSD. *Frontiers in Psychiatry, 4,* 118.

Chapter 3

Culturally Responsive Trauma-Informed Psychotherapy

Prior to introducing any therapeutic approach, the therapist must learn, listen to, and support the client's trauma narrative. This provides both the foundation for all subsequent work and an opportunity for the therapist and client to foster a safe and trusting therapeutic alliance. In my practice with BIPOC clients who are reprocessing trauma, somatic experiencing approaches have been most successful in creating rapport. Somatic experiencing was developed and founded by Dr. Peter Levine (2015); it attempts to alleviate symptoms by comprehending trauma at the cerebral/nervous system level and connecting clients to different parts of themselves. An individual who is feeling disconnected may dissociate as a form of coping, as doing so allows them to escape to seek safety and comfort within. When in a state of dissociation, it is challenging for some individuals to manage and regulate emotions and body sensations as well as process and heal from trauma. Unprocessed trauma may show up in one's body as headaches, sleep disruption, fatigue, gastrointestinal concerns, heart disease, respiratory challenges, and chronic pain issues (Levine, 1997; Maté & Maté, 2022).

Effective somatic experiencing for BIPOC could include acknowledging body sensations; titration; pendulation; grounding techniques/glimmers/self-soothing exercises; resourcing (accessing inner resilience and safety in one's mind and body, envisioning a calm and safe place); resting (to ensure one's body feels safe and is able to recover); body scans; systematic desensitization; re-evaluating and shifting belief systems; crafted exposure therapy; centring; breathing exercises; *mapping* autonomic nervous system states (e.g., ventral vagal, sympathetic, and dorsal vagal) and expanding one's window of tolerance (Siegel, 1999); and understanding emotions within the polyvagal ladder, as shown in Figure 3.1 (Dana, 2021; Dana & Porges, 2018). Created by Dan Siegel (1999), the window of tolerance is used to navigate the autonomic nervous system and balance emotions; it depicts a place where individuals feel centred, grounded, and present and can operate in their everyday life in a more emotionally regulated

DOI: 10.4324/9781003216568-5

manner. Expanding upon an individual's window of tolerance is essential to remain in the ventral vagal state, where one can feel connected, engaged, calm, and content.

Figure 3.1 is an example of a personalized version of the autonomic nervous system ladder that I use in my practice with clients. It is adapted from complex trauma specialist Deb Dana's research (2018, 2021).

Throughout all stages of therapy, I apply titration, a strategy which allows clients to slowly reprocess the trauma (Levine, 1997). During titration, clients pace themselves by sharing moment by moment while resting and pausing, allowing the work to process in their bodies, and then revisit the unresolved and contained trauma. By utilizing titration, the client may

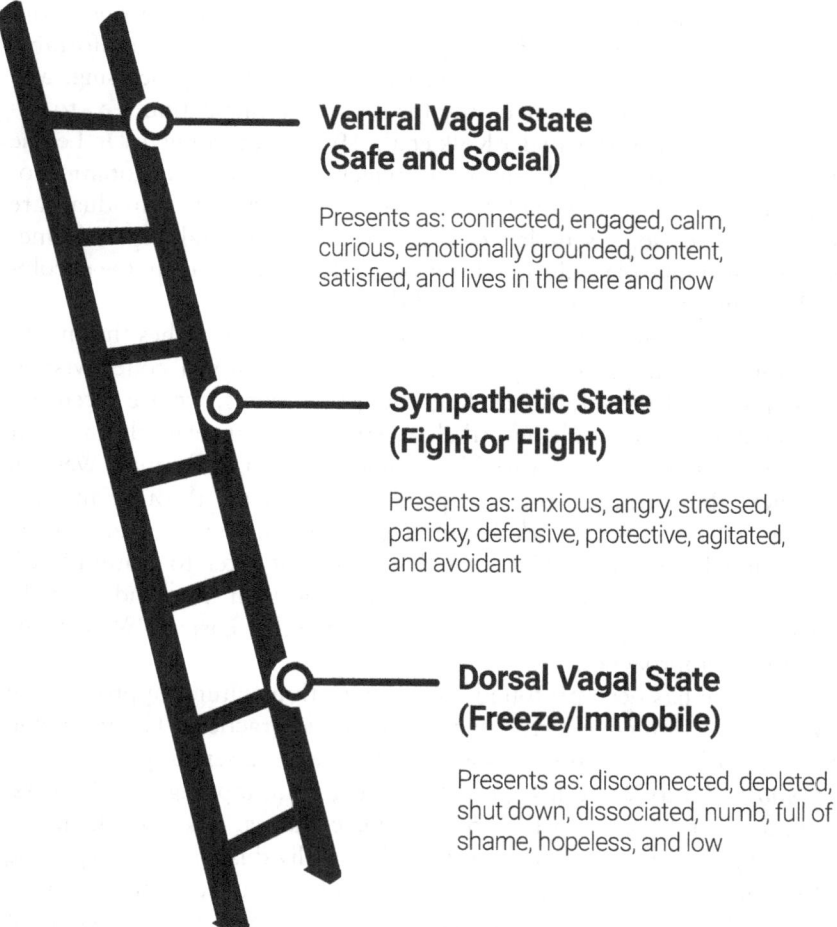

**Ventral Vagal State
(Safe and Social)**

Presents as: connected, engaged, calm, curious, emotionally grounded, content, satisfied, and lives in the here and now

**Sympathetic State
(Fight or Flight)**

Presents as: anxious, angry, stressed, panicky, defensive, protective, agitated, and avoidant

**Dorsal Vagal State
(Freeze/Immobile)**

Presents as: disconnected, depleted, shut down, dissociated, numb, full of shame, hopeless, and low

Figure 3.1 Autonomic nervous system ladder

not feel hurried to disclose their story, unlike in Western psychotherapeutic practices, where there may be some form of urgency to collect background information for diagnostic purposes (Sodhi, 2023). Clients are supported as they honour and recognize how much their body can process and prevent overwhelming their biology (Curran, 2013; MacIntosh, 2014). "It is our biology that shapes our experiences of safety and connection" (Dana, 2021, p. 13). Similar to practicing yoga, during trauma work clients are asked to pause and pivot when there are feelings of discomfort and hurt. If dissociation occurs, the client can self-regulate, prevent affect dysregulation, contend with somatic responses, expand their window of tolerance, and thus actively participate in therapy.

Titration offers the option to unpack one's trauma on a gradual basis, process/reprocess trauma, build a strong basis for reframing one's core beliefs, become empowered, feel respected, and therefore feel comfortable to share within a safe clinical space. Ultimately, safety, processing, and healing are imperative to reduce any form of retraumatization (i.e., to experience trauma again) (van der Kolk et al., 1996). According to Dr. Levine (2015), "pain is a trapped sensation" which requires a renegotiation of sorts and should not be rushed. By releasing pain and hurt, individuals are moving towards some semblance of healing. Increased stability and inner resiliency also take place during this process. This is outlined in the decolonized therapeutic techniques section of this chapter.

It should be highlighted that psychotherapeutic approaches that might work for one individual may not necessarily work on a collectivist or community level (Sodhi, 2022). Regarding treatments, we are often impressionable and hopeful; nevertheless, strategic change needs to occur for each client, and several variables should be taken in account. Western constructs about trauma might be perceived differently through an Eastern lens. This is most remarkable in assessments that are not completely intersectional, lack inclusivity, and clearly do not cater to culturally diverse demographics. Therapists must understand their own and their client's intersectionality and capacity to engage in either Eastern, Western, or decolonized approaches.

Alas, there has been profound commodification/cultural appropriation of various Eastern collectivist psychotherapeutic practices. The following principles originating from Eastern wisdom were essentially *stolen* and *commodified* into Western approaches: yoga, reiki, tapping, mindfulness, meditation, and narrative therapy. By not crediting, acknowledging, or referencing the origins of these approaches, individuals are disrespecting and discounting the value and meaning behind these beliefs and ideologies (Bruce, 2019; Cohen, 2021). As decolonial practitioners, we are on a quest to reclaim these approaches and remind the Western capitalist orientations about the integrity of these ancestral healing practices.

Therapy requires personalization in which cultural gradations *need* and *should* be taken into consideration. There is a pending need to decolonize aspects within the field of psychotherapy: accessing help, safe spaces, attachment styles, forms of dissociation, trauma responses, inner child wounds, regulation/dysregulation, and eurocentric therapeutic approaches. Clients are supported as they identify traumatic moments and events and are heard and held instead of being silenced. Trauma treatment assists in overcoming hopelessness, paranoia, and cultural mistrust. Clients are guided to lean into their spirituality, feel empowered, and connect with their cultural/ethnic/racial background, family, and community. Long-term healing innately takes place through connection.

The next part of this section shares a centralized list of decolonized therapeutic techniques.

Decolonizing Therapeutic Techniques

Any therapeutic treatment plan generally involves a myriad of recommended techniques. My Western training imparted little knowledge and instruction regarding working with multicultural clients; however, my lived BIPOC and clinical experiences have culminated in the following curated approaches to working with BIPOC clients. These techniques help practitioners understand the cultural aspect to treatment that traditional Western psychotherapeutic practices overlook. Upon determining efficacy, I posted some of these approaches on my professional Instagram platform *Suno Therapy* and received positive feedback from other BIPOC therapists. I have intentionally reduced the strategic complexity and Western language within these therapeutic methods, as such language can create barriers for BIPOC clients.

Western approaches to treating trauma often omit the concepts of holism or healing. Experiencing any form of trauma requires relinquishing suffering (Kornfield, 2008; Tirch et al., 2016). Suffering may take the form of anger, anxiety, grieving, or mourning. Comparable to trauma, suffering can be classified under Big S (Suffering) and little s (suffering) depending on the time required to heal from it. Healing may take months, years, or could be a lifelong process. Renouncing one's suffering clears the path for further healing. In addition to these decolonized methods, clients are guided to ground and journal their daily thoughts in a resiliency diary. This may evolve into somatic writing (i.e., track, notice, and comment upon their body sensation(s)) or speaking to one's ancestors for guidance. Alongside daily journalling, clients welcome psychoeducation, application of techniques/approaches (e.g., affirmations), and processing and discussing technique application, all of which will lead to gradual progress.

Circling back to polyvagal theory, resourcing oneself within a calm place is a reminder that one's nervous system is shifting and healing by means of glimmers. Dana (2018) suggests glimmers ("sparks of joy") are the opposite of emotional triggers. Triggers can activate stress/trauma responses such as fight, flight, freeze, or fawn and dysregulate one's nervous system; conversely, glimmers provide opportunities to feel safe, connected, and regulated. Examples of glimmers are connecting with nature, receiving a hug from a loved one, and the aroma of freshly brewed coffee, which are further noted in Table 3.1 (Dana, 2021).

A series of decolonized techniques, discussion points, structured activities, and experiential exercises have resonated well with my clientele. In my work with BIPOC, it goes beyond clients showing up for session; clients are invited to complete work between sessions, rest, ground, regulate, reflect, reframe, play, and apply strategies to the best of their ability. We are attempting to achieve longevity versus a temporary solution and to combine that longevity with monumental reflections that may appear after their departure from therapy.

Reclaiming Cultural Narratives

Two recurring themes within my practice are recounting past cultural narratives and unpacking present cultural narratives. Clients describe narratives about unresolved trauma and its influence on their adult mindset. I provide information about inner child work/trauma dialogue; grieving; healing; processing internalized systemic oppression; familial dynamics; interpersonal conflict; attachment styles; transference; notion of instability; boundary violations; and supportive coping strategies for clients to make sense of their dichotomies. The main intention of this phase of therapy is for clients to renarrate their story by holding space for themselves and implementing concepts such as forgiveness for self and others, self-compassion, and loving kindness in their way of being.

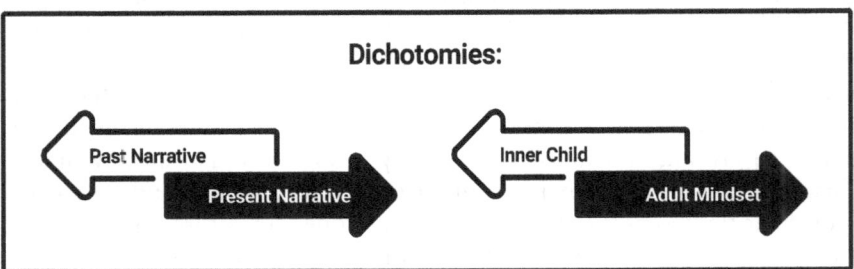

Figure 3.2 Reclaiming cultural narratives

Inner BIPOC Child Wounds

How do we address healing inner child trauma with BIPOC individuals? I have noticed with my clientele that BIPOC rarely access help to heal inner child trauma. When healing inner child trauma, it is important to discuss these vulnerabilities by envisioning "inner children" representing different parts of one's life. Inner child work allows individuals to cope better with loss, abandonment, and childhood trauma. How is inner child work different for BIPOC individuals? Themes that have arisen in my practice are cultural values and traditions, confusion around grief, love languages, safety, and trust.

It is essential to explore inner BIPOC child wounds that could be misrepresented or misinterpreted by the host culture. For example, is an immigrant parent working night shifts to make ends meet a form of abandonment? Other relevant topics worth discussing are cultural expectations versus core beliefs, the overlap between attachment styles and inner child wounds, trauma versus cultural expectations, and attachment styles based on intergenerational trauma. What has the client internalized as opposed to compartmentalized? That is, what have they suppressed instead of catalogued to resolve later?

Trauma-Healing Continuum

The continuum in Figure 3.3 structures discourse about a traumatic event. First, the client is supported while they process a traumatic event and explore stages of grief. Clients are then invited to compartmentalize and break cycles by grounding and reframing, fostering growth (and revelations), moving towards acceptance (or making room for the

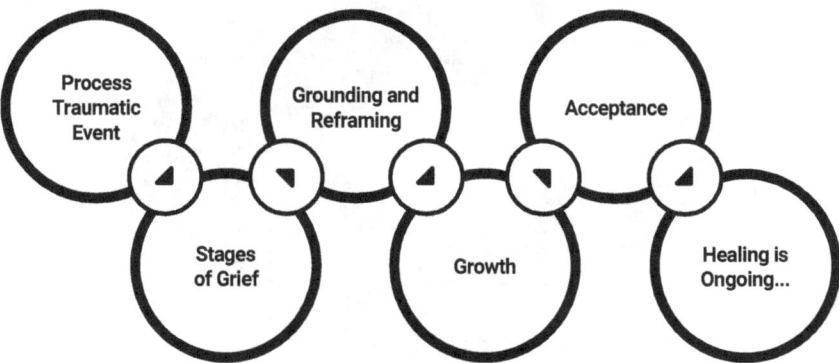

Figure 3.3 Trauma-healing continuum

experience to become a part of their psyche), determining the psychological gradient for healing, and recognizing that healing (micro or macro) is ongoing and non-linear. During this time, somatic responses may (re)surface accompanied by intrusive thoughts that could warrant either more processing or grounding.

Individual/Family Trauma Framework

Within a collectivist culture, it is possible that one's personal identity and trauma narrative is enmeshed with their family's identity and trauma narrative. This exercise demonstrates how clients can extricate their trauma from their family's trauma.

Clients complete Figure 3.4 prompts to determine overlap, learn how it is linked to their intersectionality, and further understand the rationale for internalizing familial burdens. Here are some suggestions for prompts: What individual traumas did you encounter in your life? Describe trauma that occurred within your family. What were some familial expectations? How did you internalize familial legacy burdens?

The essence of this activity is to identify the distinctness of these traumas, to externalize past shame and guilt associated with ancestral trauma, and to ascertain that these traumas are part of one's epigenetics, and that cycles can be broken with perseverance and patience in a safe space.

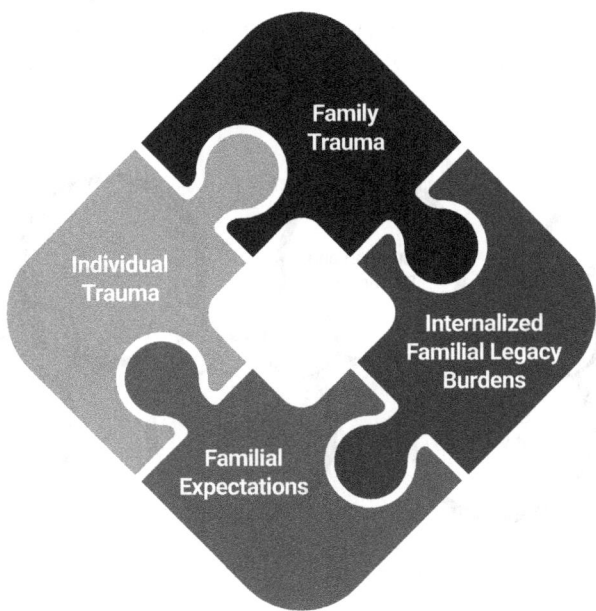

Figure 3.4 Individual/family trauma framework

Intersectional Healing

Intersectional healing is fundamental in decentring whiteness and cultivating solidarity amongst BIPOC community members (Sodhi, 2021; Tuck & Yang, 2012). By highlighting the needs, experiences, and ancestral or intergenerational barriers of the client, therapists can offer relevant approaches for long-term healing and growth. Healing as a community might entail the following:

- Nurturing togetherness, engaging in meditation and prayer to feel grounded, and reframing negative thoughts to mitigate long-term mental health effects of collective trauma.
- Supporting and justifying feelings of hypervigilance, confusion, grief, remorse, fear, low self-esteem, mistrust, and anger resulting from constant and unresolved global collective trauma.
- Facilitating meaningful conversations and/or panels about the effect of collective trauma on one's self-perception as well as interactions with members of the Western culture.

In 2021, I was invited as a panelist at the *Parliament of the World Religions* virtual conference. Our collective presentation explored "The Sikh Spirit of Chardi Kala (Resilience) as a Cure for Grief." The Sikh definition of *Chardi Kala* manifests hope, optimism, positivity, high spirits, and a visionary mindset, while "rising above adversity during difficult or challenging times." *Chardi Kala* is a way of life that emphasizes meaning and purpose while simultaneously navigating unpredictability during one's lifetime and attaining inner peace. *Chardi Kala* suggests that we acknowledge, learn, validate, and move forward from challenging events (Kaur, 2021).

For my panel contribution, I spoke about collective trauma, grief, and suffering resulting from hate crimes and racism and, in particular, the role of *Chardi Kala* in the healing process. I reinforced that the global Sikh community continues to be underrepresented in media coverage, especially in terms of trauma-related events, which necessitates being further resilient and embracing the *Chardi Kala* mantra. Figure 3.5 was created to demonstrate steps towards actualizing resiliency:

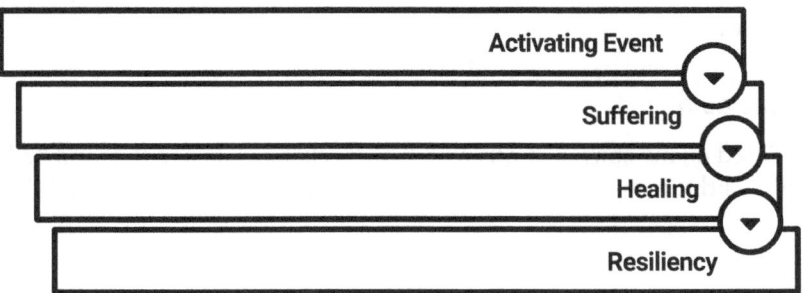

Figure 3.5 Resiliency model

The model begins with an activating event related to racism (e.g., collective trauma or a hate crime). In the next phase of the model, I ask clients the following questions: how does suffering show up in their lives? How would they liberate themselves from unnecessary suffering which intersects past suffering with current suffering? How would they process this suffering as a collective community (Denov et al., 2019; Kazlauskas et al., 2017)? The client will have a sense of being connected; if one person is suffering, community will suffer together (Sodhi, 2017; Tirch et al., 2016). The next set of inquiries are: how does one move towards healing and reconciling with this suffering? How would one adopt a resiliency mindset? BIPOC who heal rise above challenges such as racism or other white supremist acts of violence, and learn to become a stronger and complete collective unit.

Situational Grief

During the COVID-19 pandemic, I tried to understand how global and/or personal events or circumstances continue to influence my daily mood. I was finally able to name it as *situational grief*. I wondered if this term even existed. What does it entail? One way of articulating this term is as an in-between state: hoping a situation will improve over time while simultaneously experiencing non-linear stages of grief. On some occasions, the final stage of acceptance is sometimes lacking. Other manifestations of situational grief are racial violence/hate crimes, migrating to a new country, familial estrangement, and chronic mental health conditions.

By sitting and then contending with emotions related to situational grief, one can avoid severe depression or trauma-related responses. In my work with specific BIPOC clients who are tentative about actualizing the acceptance stage, we explore options around self-forgiveness, self-compassion, and subscribing to loving kindness via grief journaling prompts (e.g., Why am I grieving . . . My most cherished memory is . . . I wish I could forgive myself for . . . My grief support system is . . .). There may not be defined closure at this point in therapy, yet clients do have a clearer understanding of how these events affect their psyche and have strategies to move forward in their lives.

Ethnic Guilt

Based on my conversations with BIPOC clients, I coined the term "ethnic guilt." Ethnic guilt is typically experienced by a BIPOC individual during their interactions with parents, family (immediate or extended), and community. The feeling of guilt can be complex, and in this context, it is presented in a linear (possibly cyclical) process. Clients may start by examining the defining features:

- A fear of offending
- People pleasing tendencies
- Needing to over compromise
- Sacrificing inner happiness
- Experiencing feelings of inadequacy

Clients may fluctuate between demonstrating complacency and resentment about their thoughts and actions until they receive validation for putting others before themselves. Further exploration of past narratives allows clients to comprehend that ethnic guilt could be intergenerational, as boundaries and assertiveness may have been non-existent among previous generations. The work does not stop here; however, it is a starting point where clients can unlearn patterns and relearn strategies that would be beneficial in putting their needs first.

Stages of Forgiveness

The concept of forgiveness continues to be a universal theme and is represented differently across cultures (Joo et al., 2019). It is oftentimes linked to intergenerational conflict, grief and loss, and trauma-related concerns.

A description of the stages of forgiveness is:

- Awareness of diverse systems of thinking.
- Acknowledgement of what is unjust and hurtful.
- Reconciliation by voicing opinions and seeking feedback from impartial support.
- Letting go by engaging in cognitive reframing and understanding the duality of the situation.
- Moving forward and learning from these experiences; actualizing a compassionate way of being.

I have used these stages of forgiveness to help clients feel unbound by these non-linear and cyclical constructs as well as navigate emotions affiliated with forgiveness. Eventually, it is hoped that clients can culminate this process by achieving self-love and inner peace.

Negotiating Boundaries Within a Cultural Space

Upon becoming assertive and setting boundaries with family and community, one simultaneously sheds and grieves a part of their cultural identity. What is reiterated in my practice is the need to exercise detachment, unlearn, and put oneself first. I encourage clients to sit with their discomfort, learn to trust their instincts, and feel safe again (Tawwab, 2021).

My BIPOC clients often voice how asserting themselves and maintaining boundaries results in them being less collectivist and more distant from their ancestral culture. In our work together, I help them "grieve" this process. Such negotiation, which resembles experiencing a loss, can be hard to accept; however, it is a pivotal step in developing a bicultural identity and creating a personalized cultural space.

Establishing boundaries within cultural conditions can take time and patience. For some, being assertive and putting up boundaries are Western characteristics. What is involved with maintaining boundaries? Within a cultural context, one may experience grief and loss when they stop people pleasing and assert themselves. Demonstrating assertiveness can be equivalent to grieving a family member. Respecting ourselves means we may lose familial connections. Here are five steps for negotiating boundaries and becoming assertive:

1. Assessment.
2. Revisit individualist and collectivist values.
3. Maintenance protocols.
4. Reframe and rebuild, nurture and grow.
5. Offer insight concerning boundary setting.

When assessing with clients, ask what boundaries were successfully conveyed in the past and which boundaries were disrespected. Identify which boundaries need to be set regarding specific people or situations. There will seemingly be a contrast between individualist and collectivist values. What may have been deemed acceptable in the host culture may not be acceptable in the ancestral country or on an intergenerational level. As a result, elements of subjugation, codependency, and enmeshment may need to be re-evaluated.

"Boundaries require maintenance" (Katherine, 2000). Set clear and assertive boundaries; if they are ignored once, it is easier for it to happen again. Strengthen boundaries by understanding the right to say no, respect for feelings, acceptance of differences, and permission for expression. Reframe and rebuild by changing perceptions and narratives about the past and how one feels about it today, and separate personal experiences from self-worth. Build boundaries by increasing self-awareness; reflect upon present boundaries in one's life. Lastly, nurture and expand upon boundaries by recognizing that boundaries can be flexible and modified in response to a situation. Boundaries are imperative, provide a clearer sense of self and relationship with others, and determine how one will be treated.

"Cultural Never Good Enough" Cycle

This framework demonstrates a cycle of never feeling good enough and the stages that often loop the client back into this scarcity mindset. This exercise is inspired by my BIPOC clients' voices and the associated suggestions I offer to break the "Cultural Never Good Enough" cycle. My recommendations also originate from my dialogue with clients who try to be enough. Fueled by capitalist and patriarchal ideologies, the core beliefs of never being good enough can arise in individuals who are constantly

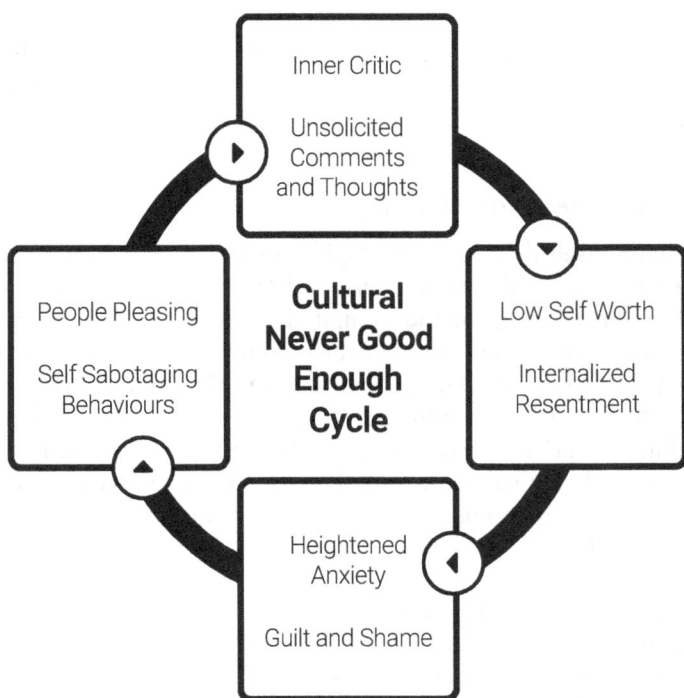

Figure 3.6 Cultural never good enough cycle

striving, or present as overachievers, perfectionists, trauma survivors, or those who over compromise in various aspects of their life.

The proceeding list offers viable suggestions for unlearning and breaking this cycle and replacing it with ways of elevating one's self-esteem and self-worth:

- Make yourself a priority.
- Practice self-compassion.
- Heal inner child wounds.
- Take social media breaks.
- Let go of perfectionist tendencies.
- Celebrate ALL your accomplishments.
- Become assertive and set boundaries.
- Surround yourself with positive and supportive people.
- Shift from a scarcity mindset to an abundance mindset.
- Access inner resources such as self-love and self-respect; negate self-judgement.
- Relinquish culturally ingrained messaging and rewrite past narratives.

I invite clients to replace these deeply embedded core beliefs with positive messaging, nurture a more secure sense of self, and therefore actualize being more than enough.

Silencing the Inner Cultural Critic

The inner cultural critic can be highly pronounced in BIPOC. It can be a combination of family expectations and self-expectations, or shame and blame for not adhering to indoctrinated cultural and family traditions, values, and beliefs. What arises in turn from the inner critic are feelings of inadequacy when comparing oneself to family and the ethnic community, which then devolves into anxiety, panic attacks, and/or depression. Succumbing to the inner critic may result in a freeze trauma response in which one might be silenced, immobilized due to the harshness of their inner critic, or of the opinion that they exhibit imposter syndrome. These strategies may help:

1. Engage in inner child imagery.
2. Write the inner child a letter.
3. Recognize patterns and somatically process.
4. Assert oneself in a familial, work, and/or community context.
5. Understand the origins of the inner critic voice: whose voice is it? Mother, sister, self? Is it an intergenerational inner critic?

These methods may tame one's inner critic and lead a more authentic and liberated life. No one deserves to be spoken to or silenced in this manner.

Culturally Relevant Trauma Responses

During my therapeutic conversations with BIPOC clients, as we gradually co-construct their narratives, it is apparent that different trauma responses surface when they try to actualize cultural ideals. Consistently, these reactions occur in response to interactions with family and community.

Figure 3.7 outlines how I have witnessed common trauma responses manifest in my BIPOC clients.

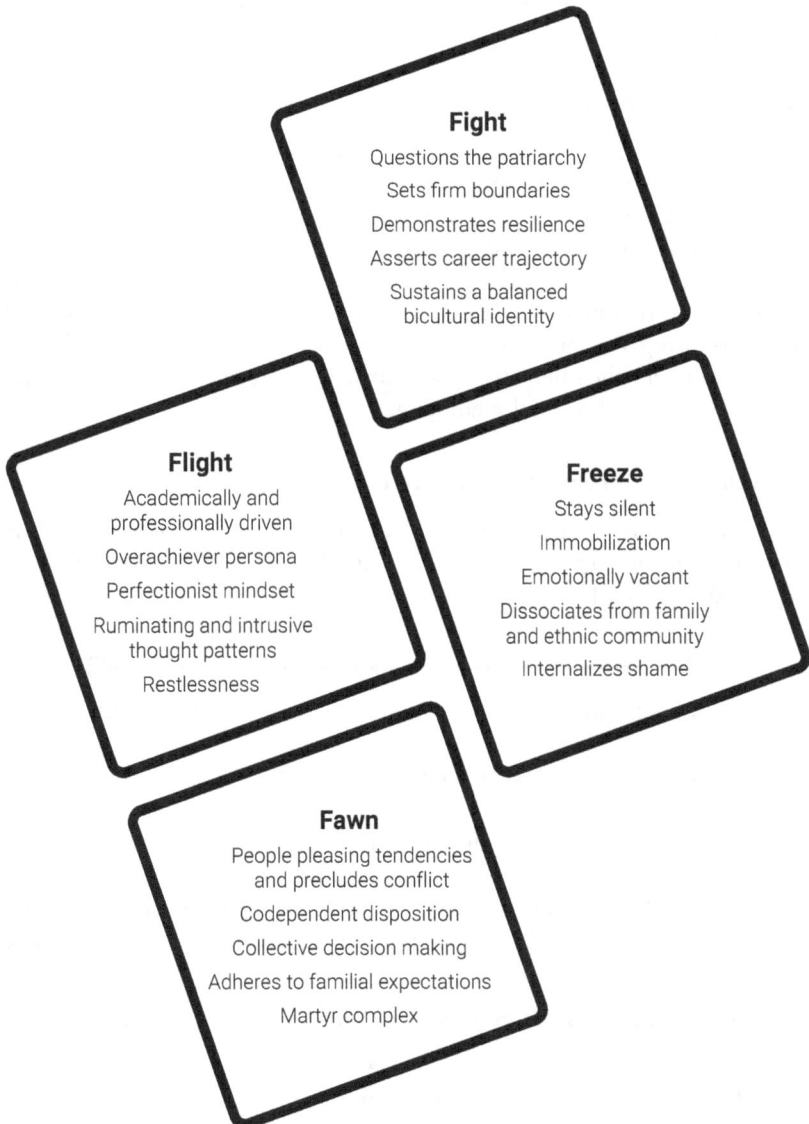

Figure 3.7 Culturally relevant trauma responses

Please note the following about Figure 3.7:

- Collectivist language and ideologies are included.
- Cultural expectations are distinguished from trauma responses.
- Discern the language chosen to describe each trauma response.
- Recognize that urgency and overexplaining are overlooked trauma responses.

The duality of each trauma response should be acknowledged; what might be considered unsuitable in one culture is lauded in another, causing conflict within the BIPOC psyche.

Cultural Safety Road Map

In a safe space, co-contruct the client's original trauma road map. Then compose the re-narrated cultural safety road map, which includes steps to prevent retraumatization by grounding, unlearning, reframing, and desensitization practices. Afterwards, compare the original trauma road map with the renarrated cultural safety road map and explore barriers and triumphs within this process. The aim of this exercise is for the client to feel safe by treating the problem, rather than the symptomology. This technique empowers the client to make conscious decisions and take a stance toward overall healing and wellbeing.

Codependent-Interdependent Spectrum

In recent family-related work, to learn more about a client's attachment style and relationship with family, I created this spectrum (see Figure 3.8) and asked clients where they land:

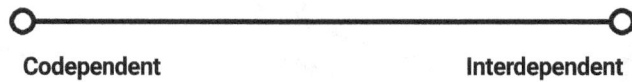

Codependent   **Interdependent**

Figure 3.8 Codependent-interdependent spectrum

The intention is to encourage clients to move from a codependent identity to an interdependent identity. Further conversation about subjugation, boundary setting, and becoming assertive ensue. As well, I ask clients "How do these shifts occur?" and "What is being preserved and what is being let go?"

Grounding Techniques, Glimmers, and Self-Soothing Exercises

This exercise asks clients to list the grounding techniques, glimmers, and self-soothing exercises that resonate with them. Examples of each of the following are listed in Table 3.1.

Table 3.1 Grounding techniques, glimmers, and self-soothing exercises

Grounding Techniques	Glimmers	Self-Soothing Exercises
• breathwork • mindful walking • affirmations • singing • tapping • touching something hot or cold • having a glass of water • hand on the heart • meditation • movement/exercise • listening to music or sound • body scans • humming • cherishing and holding a safe grounding object	• holding a hand • noticing a smile or kind gestures • connecting with nature • hearing a favourite song on a playlist • watching a sunset • looking at photos of loved ones or favourite places • playing with a pet • admiring the stars in the sky • seeing a rainbow • the aroma of freshly brewed coffee	• taking a warm shower • relaxing to calming music • nourishing oneself with favourite foods • change of environment • petting an animal • focusing on self-compassion • wearing comfortable clothing • resting • feeling one's feelings

By documenting and/or tracking the efficacy of different grounding techniques, glimmers, and self-soothing exercises, clients identify what they can refer to during activating events.

This part of the book offers a comprehensive account of trauma-informed content. This awareness sets the stage for the rest of the book as we explore deconstructing racism, listening to BIPOC narratives, and most importantly, navigating clinical implications.

References

Bruce, R. D. (2019). White supremacist yoga: A black feminist perspective on cultural appropriation. *Systemic*, 16.

Cohen, E. (2021). *The psychologisation of eastern spiritual traditions: Colonisation, translation and commodification.* Routledge.

Curran, L. (2013). *101 Trauma-informed interventions: Activities, exercises and assignments to move the client and therapy forward.* Premier Publishing and Media.

Dana, D. (2018). *The polyvagal theory in therapy: Engaging the rhythm of regulation.* W. W. Norton.

Dana, D. (2021). *Anchored: How to befriend your nervous system using polyvagal theory.* Sound True.

Dana, D., & Porges, S. W. (2018). *The polyvagal theory in therapy: Engaging the rhythm of regulation.* W.W. Norton & Company.

Denov, M., Fennig, M., Rabiau, M. A., & Shevell, M. C. (2019). Intergenerational resilience in families affected by war, displacement, and migration: "It runs in the family". *Journal of Family Social Work*, 22(1), 17–45.

Joo, M., Terzino, K. A., Cross, S. E., Yamaguchi, N., & Ohbuchi, K.-I. (2019). How does culture shape conceptions of forgiveness? Evidence from Japan and the United States. *Journal of Cross-Cultural Psychology, 50*(5), 67, 6–702.

Katherine, A. (2000). *Where to draw the line: How to set healthy boundaries every day*. Fireside.

Kaur, V. (2021). *See no stranger: A memoir and manifesto of revolutionary love*. One World.

Kazlauskas, E., Gailiene, D., Vaskeliene, I., & Skeryte-Kazlauskiene, M. (2017). Intergenerational transmission of resilience? Sense of coherence is associated between Lithuanian survivors of political violence and their adult offspring. *Frontiers in Psychology, 8*, 1677, 1–8.

Kornfield, J. (2008). *The art of forgiveness, lovingkindness, and peace*. Bantam Books.

Levine, P. A. (1997). *Waking the tiger: Healing trauma*. North Atlantic Books.

Levine, P. A. (2015). *Trauma and memory: Brain and body in a search for the living past: A practical guide for understanding and working with traumatic memory*. North Atlantic Books.

MacIntosh, H. B. (2014). Titration of technique: Clinical exploration of the integration of trauma model and relational psychoanalytic approaches to the treatment of dissociative identity disorder. *Psychoanalytic Psychology, 32*, 517–538.

Maté, G., & Maté, D. (2022). *The myth of normal: Trauma, illness, and healing in a toxic culture*. Knopf Canada.

Siegel, D. J. (1999). *The developing mind: How relationships and the brain interact to shape who we are*. The Guilford Press.

Sodhi, P. K. (2017). *Exploring immigrant and sexual minority mental health: Reconsidering multiculturalism*. Routledge.

Sodhi, P. K. (2021). The Sikh spirit of Chardi Kala (resilience) as a cure for grief. Panelist. *Parliament of the World's Religions virtual conference*, October 16–18, 2021.

Sodhi, P. K. (2022). Trauma-informed care for BIPOC communities. Speaker series hosted by the *Canadian Counselling and Psychotherapy Association*, November 16, 2022.

Sodhi, P. K. (2023). Trauma-informed approaches for current and future lawyers. Webinar presented to the *Women's Legal Mentorship Program*, Ottawa, Ontario, January 26, 2023.

Tawwab, N. G. (2021). *Set boundaries, find peace: A guide to reclaiming yourself*. TarcherPerigee.

Tirch, D., Siberstein, L. R., & Kolts, R. L. (2016). *Buddhist psychology and cognitive-behavioral therapy*. The Guilford Press.

Tuck, E., & Yang, W. K. (2012). Decolonization is not a metaphor. *Decolonization: Indigeneity, Education & Society, 1*(1), 1–40.

van der Kolk, B. A., MacFarlane, A. C., & Weisaeth, L. (Eds.). (1996). *Traumatic stress: The effects of overwhelming experience on mind, body and society*. The Guilford Press.

Part 2

Deconstructing Systemic Racism

Introduction

Racism supports a white colonial unified initiative and consists of four foundations: prejudice, oppression, white privilege, and white supremacy. Colonial racism commenced centuries before slavery and segregation; its origins were rooted in the "ideologies of class" instead of nationalism (Anderson, 2006; Haque, 2012). It can be traced back to the discordant interactions between different religious and cultural groups over 600 years ago and the need for power and exclusive domination (Davis,1983; Kendi, 2019). The first documented racist person dates back to 1415: Prince Henry, who captured a Muslim trading depot due to pure envy of their wealth (Kendi, 2016). This is an example of the kind of interactions that yield biases and beliefs about certain groups. These exchanges enable mistreatment of disenfranchised racialized communities and render complicit acts of shame and humiliation acceptable. More and more therapy-based research is suggesting the importance of anti-racist positioning within the therapeutic space (Hook et al., 2016; Ratts, 2017). As a BIPOC psychotherapist, I would like to share a personal narrative, titled *The Cultural Elephant in the Room*, that I wrote after experiencing a common microaggression from a client (Abrams, 2018; Ahmed et al., 2011; Badwall, 2014; Constantine, 2007).

> *As we collectively raise awareness around anti-racist causes, it is important to implement relevant approaches in our clinical practices. The cultural elephant in the room can consist of, but is not exclusive to, microaggressions, cultural ignorance, shadeism, internalized colourism, generalized racial stereotypes, and covert racism that occurs within the therapeutic space (or any space, for that matter). Clients are generally at the receiving end of culturally inappropriate comments. However, as a psychotherapist, I have experienced uneasiness and discomfort while navigating this familiar territory.*

DOI: 10.4324/9781003216568-6

During the summer of 2020, a client asked me, "Where are you from?" It has been over a decade since I have been asked this question, so I decided to frame my response as a teachable moment for the client. I said, "I was born in Canada." She looked at me with confusion, so I added, "My parents are originally from India." I then asked her if she was familiar with the culture, and she said no. I decided to share what I have learned about the culture (e.g., Eastern worldviews such as self-compassion, loving kindness) and how this informs my practice. These details resonated with her and offered a piece of cultural knowledge that she was not aware of prior to working with me. I believe discussing her inquiry strengthened the therapeutic alliance.

The same method (i.e., reflecting, exploring one's worldviews, and linking my response to my therapeutic approach) can be applied if a client makes a racist remark about a cultural group or labels a cultural group in a derogatory manner. The unlearning and relearning dialogue can begin by asking the client their understanding of the culture, exploring the history of the cultural group, and concluding by reminding the client of this population's contribution to society.

As therapists shift towards becoming more anti-racist practitioners, every teachable moment is necessary to eradicate systemic and structural racism and educate others on the importance of being empathic and respectful to humankind.

I added further reflections on racism on January 19, 2021, the eve of the US Presidential Inauguration, which seemed appropriate at the time. Irrespective of the efforts to mitigate systemic racism and cultural stereotypes, we continue to live in a world where cultural responsiveness and inclusivity are constantly being challenged by select members of our global society. During a conversation with a colleague, we discussed our work with clients, specifically regarding professional and personal values. The topic of cultural curiosity was examined in terms of building a solid therapeutic alliance with our clients. Unfortunately, cultural ignorance can also be present within one's therapeutic setting and Western culture. My definitions are noted below:

> **Cultural curiosity entails sincere, authentic inquiring or clarifying about an individual's cultural background. It is an opportunity to learn and develop a deeper understanding of one's knowledge concerning multicultural topics.**

> **Cultural ignorance occurs when individuals demonstrate a lack of understanding towards another's cultural background. It can involve interrogating, negotiating, and judging one's beliefs and values and/ or having disrespectful opinions about culturally related matters.**

The topic of my ethnicity has been brought up in either a cultur-ally curious or culturally ignorant manner by my clients. In the past, I would admittedly become defensive or reinforce the fact that I am a second-generation immigrant (so really not from my ancestral country). I have learned over the years that I internalized these covert microag-gressions and was not being true to my personal values. I typically felt uncomfortable and remorseful for these actions and therefore decided the next time this occurred with a client, I would address this topic in a compassionate manner (hence the reflection about the cultural elephant in the room). These therapeutic incidents transpire as an inquiry about a therapist's cultural background, worldview, or any multicultural con-cept. This is one way of implementing anti-racist awareness and decolo-nizing our practices with prospective clients.

Similarly, DiAngelo (2018) expresses:

While speaking up against these explicitly racist actions is critical, we must also be careful not to use them to keep ourselves on the "good" side of a false binary. I have found it much more useful to think of myself as on a continuum. Racism is so deeply woven into the fabric of society that I do not see myself escaping from that continuum in my lifetime. But I can continually seek to move further along it. I am not in a fixed position on the continuum; my position is dictated by what I am actually doing at a given time.

(p. 87)

Elaborating on this belief, how can racism be reframed or unlearned? What needs to be further disrupted to preclude racism? Does this require developing an anti-racist stance?

Diverse cultures have been profoundly debilitated by global colonialism. Cultural assimilation is synonymous with colonialism. In both instances, cultural, racial, religious, and linguistic rights are taken away and replaced with Western ideologies which are somehow considered more civilized. Who determines what is appropriate for existing settlers and immigrants in a given region? Reflecting on the symbolism behind Canada Day or July 4th, I recognize that these holidays elicit different meanings depending on one's intersectionality, ancestry, time spent in the country, and what was sacrificed upon living in a colonized space. Currently, many such eurocen-tric and imperialist "celebrations" are being scrutinized and cancelled due to their obsolescence and derogation of BIPOC, who internalize racism and negative cultural perception of self from these colonized events.

Ijeoma Oluo (2019) asserted, "When we acknowledge racism as a part of a system, instead of being limited to our ability to win over racists, we can instead focus on how our actions interact with systemic racism." There is a distinct overlap between my personal and professional lives. In addition to personally reading and relating to content from Ijeoma Oluo's book, *So you Want to Talk about Race* (2019), my family and friends have fear-driven conversations about colonization, everyday racism, feeling othered, and being a potential target of hate crime. No matter how much we condemn racists, active racism will continue to be omnipresent unless we name and decentre instead of normalizing it. How would our ancestors respond to this current day oppression? Would they encourage accessible dialogue, messaging, and education concerning inclusion and diversity? Meanwhile, BIPOC will protect themselves from the next microaggression, hate crime, police brutality . . . until someone stops silencing them and hears their voices.

Ibram Kendi (2019) likens racism to cancer and posits that by using conventional (anti-racist) treatments, we can in fact eradicate racism. Surgery can remove cancerous tumours, and chemotherapy is another treatment option, but parallel to racism, the issue is more systemic. Conventional strategies to excise racism may be temporary and representative of performative allyship. How can we ultimately get to the root of the issue and understand why some people are racist? We need to be creative with our anti-racist approaches so that the individual produces long-term results. Should one look beyond conventional or standardized methods and understand how racism is conceptualized and stored in the brain? There are other systemic causes, too: emotional, environmental, lifestyle, and dietary factors can breed anger that may become displaced onto other racial demographics. James Baldwin (1984) expressed, "I imagine one of the reasons people cling to their hate so stubbornly is because they sense, once the hate is gone, they will be forced to deal with pain" (p. 104); perhaps the link between racism and hate could broaden our awareness on self-perception and magnifying pain?

Different types of racism have happened, are happening, and will happen. How do we further understand and prepare ourselves to be at the receiving end of these various forms of racism? The first step involves learning what causes an individual to become racist and the impact racism has on their brain.

How Does One Become Racist?

It is a known fact that our brains are capable of simultaneously storing both necessary and trivial information either in our working memory, short-term memory, or long-term memory. We can also seemingly discard information until it resurfaces later. Hinged on an individual's lived experience, there is an emotional link between the content that is stored in the brain and whether this content emerges in other contexts. This is true of all members of society when we develop stereotypes, prejudices, judgment, and biases towards other cultural/ethnic/racial groups (Bailey et al., 2021; Greer & Dixon, 2020).

These race-related messages indeed start at a young age and are often influenced by a person's ecosystems: home, academic setting, community, and host culture. In essence, culture affects our way of being (Salter et al., 2018). That is, throughout our lifetime, we are internalizing messages about race, storing them in our brains, and constantly forming opinions towards other cultural/ethnic/racial groups. Over time, these unconscious biases about race are layered with other memories which in turn perpetuate and embed these attitudes and judgments about race within our mindset (Eberhardt, 2019; Feagin, 2013). Unconscious bias programs the brain to create unsound racial opinions, hatred, and hidden beliefs stemming from past experiences and situations and subsequently impacts the way we process thoughts and behaviours. These forms of biases are usually directed towards minoritized demographics (Canadian Human Rights Act, 2021; Crenshaw, 2022), as mentioned in this passage:

> I often have fascinating conversations with BIPOC individuals about racism. I spoke with my physiotherapist who is originally from Kerala, India, regarding COVID-19 related stereotypes and fears about the "India Variant." She shared microaggressions directed towards her due to the misunderstandings about the Delta and Delta+ variant. She was asked by patients if she will be travelling to India or if her family is planning to visit her. She felt compelled to reassure her patients that she is not going to India for the next three years. I was able to empathize, as I too have experienced strange looks when people called the new variant the "India Variant," as if I was part of the creation of it. I was so relieved when they renamed it the Delta and Delta+ variant.

Neuroscience supports the idea that racism and racial biases can be unlearned. Doidge (2015) and Gibson (2019) both postulate that the brain can rewire, adapt, and transform thoughts associated with negative events. This occurs through neuroplasticity, which is "the ability of the nervous system to change its activity in response to intrinsic or extrinsic stimuli by reorganizing its structure, functions, or connections" (Mateos-Aparicio & Rodríguez-Moreno, 2019, p. 1). What would be required for the brain to rewire racism? And to what extent will a BIPOC's nervous system be activated before said BIPOC is able to acknowledge the necessity of reframing their biases towards racial causes and injustice?

This part of the book continues to critically examine historical and contemporary ideologies about racism, mental health implications resulting from racism, and strategies to diminish racism by developing an anti-racist stance.

References

Abrams, Z. (2018, April). When therapists face discrimination. *Monitor on Psychology, 49*(4). Retrieved August 22, 2021, from www.apa.org/monitor/2018/04/therapists-discrimination

Ahmed, S., Wilson, K. B., Henriksen, R. C., & Jones, J. W. (2011). What does it mean to be a culturally-competent counselor? *Journal for Social Action in Counseling and Psychology, 3*, 17–28.

Anderson, B. (2006). *Imagined communities*. Verso.

Badwall, H. (2014). Colonial encounters: Racialized social workers negotiating professional scripts of whiteness. *Intersectionalities: A Global Journal of Social Work Analysis, Research, Polity, and Practice, 3*, 1–21.

Bailey, Z., Feldman, J., & Bassett, M. (2021). How structural racism works – Racist policies as a root cause of U.S. racial health inequities. *New England Journal of Medicine, 384*, 768–773.

Baldwin, J. (1984). *The fire next time*. Vintage Books.

Canadian Human Rights Act. (2021). *(R.S.C., 1985, c. H-6)*. Retrieved August 27, 2021, from https://canlii.ca/t/555n8

Constantine, M. G. (2007). Racial microaggressions against African American clients in cross-racial counseling relationships. *Journal of Counseling Psychology, 54*(1), 1–16.

Crenshaw, K. (2022). *Intersectionality: Essential writings*. The New Press.

Davis, A. Y. (1983). *Women, race & class*. Vintage Books.

DiAngelo, R. (2018). *White fragility: Why it's so hard for white people to talk about racism*. Beacon Press.

Doidge, N. (2015). *The brain's way of healing: Remarkable discoveries and recoveries from the frontiers of neuroplasticity*. Penguin Books.

Eberhardt, J. L. (2019). *Biased: Uncovering the hidden prejudice that shapes what we, think, and do*. Penguin Books.

Feagin, J. (2013). *The white racial frame: Centuries of racial framing and counterframing* (2nd ed.). Routledge.

Gibson, J. R. (2019). *How racism has changed the human brain: Neuroplasticity and the chronic stress of everyday racism in contemporary America*. KITABU Publishing.

Greer, J., & Dixon, P. (2020). *Bias, racism & the brain: How we got here & what needs to happen*. OBI Press.

Haque, E. (2012). *Multiculturalism within a bilingual framework: Language, race, and belonging in Canada*. University of Toronto Press.

Hook, J. N., Farrell, J. E., Davis, D. E., DeBlaere, C., Van Tongeren, D. R., & Utsey, S. O. (2016). Cultural humility and racial microaggressions in counseling. *Journal of Counseling Psychology, 63*, 269–277.

Kendi, I. X. (2016). *Stamped from the beginning: The definitive history of racist ideas in America*. Bold Type Books.

Kendi, I. X. (2019). *How to be an antiracist*. One World.

Mateos-Aparicio, P., & Rodríguez-Moreno, A. (2019). The impact of studying brain plasticity. *Frontiers in Cellular Neuroscience, 13*(66), 1–5.

Oluo, I. (2019). *So you want to talk about race.* Seal Press.

Ratts, M. J. (2017). Charting the center and the margins: Addressing identity, marginalization, and privilege in counseling. *Journal of Mental Health Counseling, 39*(2), 87–103.

Salter, P. S., Adams, G., & Perez, M. (2018). Racism in the structure of everyday worlds: A cultural-psychological perspective. *Current Directions in Psychological Science, 27*(3), 150–155.

Chapter 4

Unpacking and Conceptualizing Racism

This chapter provides an individual overview of racism (i.e., origins of structural and systemic racism), critical race theory, systems of oppression, intersectionality, capitalism, colonialism, and the patriarchy. It concludes with a framework that connects these concepts.

What Is Racism Exactly?

Racism has been prolific since the beginning of humankind and has been characterized by numerous types of sociopolitical conflict (Davis, 1983; Hogart & Fletcher, 2018; McKague, 1991). Racism emerged to racially differentiate individuals of European descent from those who had African ancestry and a history of enslavement. Soon after, it presupposed dividing, segregating, discriminating, and conquering linguistic and religious communities based on racial superiority (Shiao & Woody, 2021). There are speculations that the origins of racism commenced during the Greek and Roman times, or the Middle Ages during the "race making" era. Also noteworthy is the mistreatment of Jewish and Islamic communities and the start of slavery of these groups (Seth, 2020). Some have considered the objectivity of racism; however, the range of racist acts spans from microaggressions into more racial violence and hate crimes worldwide. Additionally, everyday racism is commonly represented via stereotyping, discrimination, and microaggressions; this is due to the unwritten power dynamics that often exist within the Western colonial culture. These messages potentially permeate within many households and academic milieus.

Racism is a multifaceted and nuanced oppressive system (DiAngelo, 2018). There are several definitions that capture the depth of racism, whether it is grounded in critical race theory (which is discussed later in this chapter) or other race-related frameworks such as the global critical race and racism (GCRR) framework (Christian, 2019). Clair and Denis (2015) suggest that in order to explicate racism, one must define race, which "was first used to describe peoples and societies in the way we

DOI: 10.4324/9781003216568-7

now understand ethnicity or national identity" (p. 857). Complementing this are Solórzano et al. (2002) (inspired by Audrey Lorde (1992)) and Manning Marable's (1992) definitions, which provide three fundamental premises of racism: "(1) one group believes itself to be superior, (2) the group that believes itself to be superior has power to carry out the racist behavior, and (3) racism affects multiple racial/ethnic groups" (p. 24).

Adding to these definitions, the impact of Western colonialism and systemic racism continues to compromise the mental health and overall wellbeing of BIPOC communities (Blue et al., 2015; Viruell-Fuentes et al., 2012):

> Systemic racism emphasizes the involvement of whole systems, and often all systems – for example, political, legal, economic, healthcare, school, and criminal justice systems – including the structures that uphold the systems. Structural racism emphasizes the role of the structures (laws, policies, institutional practices, and entrenched norms) that are the systems' scaffolding. Because systemic racism includes structural racism, for brevity we often use systemic racism to refer to both; at times we use both for emphasis. Institutional racism is sometimes used as a synonym for systemic or structural racism, as it captures the involvement of institutional systems and structures in race-based discrimination and oppression.
>
> (Braveman et al., 2022, p. 172)

BIPOC communities are seeking much deserved compassion as a result of experiencing intergenerational layers of trauma over the centuries (Kirmayer et al., 2014). Settler colonization has left an imprint; alas, earlier settlers recognized racial and cultural differences and chose to take advantage of their privilege and forced their Western ideologies, values, and beliefs on to the Indigenous communities. To this day, educational documents contain eurocentric, patriarchal, individualist, and monolingual language that clearly perpetuates the cycle and patronizes BIPOC individuals. As a BIPOC woman, I have encountered barriers in establishing an in-between space (instead of either being part of the Eastern or Western worlds) and recognizing the undertones associated with racism. There is always a starting point for experiencing racism, and rather than an end point, there is a mosaic of racist activities: microaggressions, internalized racism, hate crimes, and so on. One of my intentions in writing this book is to share my intergenerational experiences with racism:

> *My daughters and I have assorted conversations about racism. As I note in the main introduction, both daughters have experienced direct or vicarious forms of racism. The year before she began applying to*

universities, my eldest daughter shared her concerns about enrolling in select provincial institutions. She was tentative about going to a particular university due to its perceived whiteness and fear of being a target of a hate crime. She said that in her online research of her preferred university, there were only pictures of white people represented. She also talked to other racialized peers about this school who had decided not to apply due to its lack of diversity. She hopes to attend a university where she feels safe. I asked her where her fear originates from and if it stemmed back to her experiences of racism from junior kindergarten and onward (microaggressions) or if she is more aware or responsive to racism. I questioned how to reframe hypervigilance to racism if that was indeed the case for her.

Reflecting on what my daughter conveyed to me:

I did not have the luxury of choosing which university I was going to attend. My father was a professor at Dalhousie University and received reduced tuition for his children, so the decision was already made for me. Dalhousie University was a smaller yet reputable east coast school during the 1990s. There were a variety of student-led cultural groups amongst all the whiteness. Each group would showcase their culture by means of an annual or biannual cultural event. I was a member of the INDISA, the Indian Students' Association that invited individuals from the Indian subcontinent to be a part of this multifaceted group. My friends also tended to be of different cultural backgrounds. Looking back, I never felt othered, and wonder if it was a different time or if racism was simply ignored.

We are living in a space where history repeats itself and endorses white centrality and individualism (Bhatt et al., 2013; DiAngelo, 2018). To fully appreciate the affiliated messages, it is essential to explore theoretical ideologies that shape racism within today's society, explicitly critical race theory (De La Garza & Ono, 2016; Delgado & Stefancic, 2017; Hartlep, 2009) and intersectionality (Crenshaw, 1989, 1991, 2022), followed by an understanding of what capitalism, colonialism, and the patriarchy entail.

Critical Race Theory

Critical race theory (henceforth CRT) is an epistemological framework that can be used to further comprehend racial and community identity, as well as these identities' contribution towards internalized racism (Hartlep, 2009). CRT was founded by activists, including Derrick Bell, Audre Lorde, Richard Delgado, Angela Davis, and Kimberlé Crenshaw in the mid-1970s during two movements: critical legal studies and radical feminism (Bell, 1995; Delgado & Stefancic, 2017). CRT activists and scholars belonging to the movements aimed to reconcile differences between race, racism, law, and power during the critical legal studies movement and increase visibility of race-related matters in the educational system. CRT also subscribes to "how white supremacy as a legal, cultural, and political condition is reproduced and maintained, primarily in the US context" (De La Garza & Ono, 2016, p. 1). Furthermore, CRT endorses, "affirmative action policies, provision of truth with issues of urban planning (that include gentrification/segregation), and equal and fair housing rights" (Hartlep, 2009, p. 6).

Central to CRT are five notable points: (1) racism is real; the permanence of racism needs to be examined in scholarly literature, as it is an integral sociopolitical and economic component of the North American society; (2) BIPOC storytelling and narratives are told predominantly through "counter-stories" that distort BIPOC narratives regarding racial injustices; (3) only racial causes benefitting members of the white culture yield support, which is a concept called "interest convergence"; (4) critique of liberalism is rooted in the belief that there should be legal objectivity and equality towards everyone; and (5) whiteness is property insofar as only white individuals possess and have certain rights such as enjoyment, exclusion, and ownership. These five points elucidate the white supremacy cycle (Delgado & Stefancic, 2017, Frieson, 2022; Hiraldo, 2010).

In 2021, concerns and conflict arose regarding teaching CRT within the US curriculum. Some believe that American students are taught that America is racist and to discriminate against white individuals to overcome racial injustice. These states have passed legislation/CRT Bills and have chosen to remove CRT from the curriculum: Idaho, Oklahoma, Tennessee, Texas, Iowa, New Hampshire, Arizona, and South Carolina; an additional 20 states plan to follow suit (Teitelbaum, 2022).

Systems of Oppression and Intersectionality

Paolo Freire (1970) penned, "The oppressed, instead of striving for liberation, tend themselves to become oppressors." One could compare this sentiment to systemic racism, where the cycle is perpetuated by the transmission of anger, anxiety, depression, grief, stress, and sadness from one generation to the next. How can "we" as members of society empower socially constructed oppressed communities, who have been affected by colonization, racism, enslavement, wars, and genocide, grieve, break intergenerational cycles, feel liberated, and become resilient?

Systems of oppression significantly affect one's intersectionality and aptitude for learning more about the varying forms of injustice and discerning the historical patterns and trends of racial inequity and hurt. Oppression, which can be considered contrary to privilege, can manifest itself on individual and systemic levels as well as being represented in one's intersectionality (Collins & Bilge, 2016). Intersectionality, a concept developed by Kimberlé Crenshaw (1989, 1991), is defined as explicit/implicit identity related traits such as culture, ethnicity, race, religion/faith, spirituality, language, gender, gender identity, social class, sexual orientation, ability, education, and age. Three forms of intersectionality exist: structural, political, and representational. Layers of oppression entrenched in one's intersectionality considerably impact encompassing social identities and may cause suffering (Crenshaw as quoted in Steinmetz, 2020). This oppression may result in racism, sexism, classism, ableism, ageism, religious oppression, homophobia, heterosexism, and xenophobia, whereby select groups are marginalized to augment the social status in dominant groups (CRIAW, 2009).

It could be argued that examining intersectionality via *definitional fluidity* may overcome diverse forms of oppression. Being set in what defines our identity causes more conflict within one's cultural locations (Collins, 2015). Oppression, one's privilege, unwarranted power, or advantage available to a particular group of people or their intersectionality require further examination. To cope in the presence of an oppressor, one must produce a behaviour that would be approved by the oppressor. This may reduce anxiety about not fitting in but is not good for the psyche. Lastly, one's power, ability to create change or influence others via actions, communication, and relationships are imperative in determining one's disposition towards oppression (Shramko et al., 2019).

Beliefs surrounding anti-Indigenous oppression and the transformation of Indigenous individuals to non-Indigenous Canadians are deep-rooted in Canada's colonial and racist history which originates from the settlement on Aboriginal land (Fonseca, 2020). The existence of "Indian reserves" is a harsh reality of the segregation of the Indigenous communities from the Western culture (Musto, 1990). There are other forms of institutional and violent racism that Indigenous peoples encounter within the justice system, healthcare, and schools that continue to perpetuate stereotypes and labelling (Fonseca, 2020; Statistics Canada, 2021). According to Kitching et al. (2020), Indigenous communities confront racial injustices that "contribute to procedural neglect (care behaviour that falls short of the standards that constitute good care) and caring neglect (care behaviour that leads to the belief that healthcare staff 'do not care')" (p. 41). These discriminatory variables compound and worsen the mental health status of Indigenous populations, who are unable to seek ethical medical attention (Allan &Smylie, 2015; Gee & Ford, 2011; Spence et al., 2016).

Research indicates that Indigenous women living on reserves experience "lower life expectancy, elevated morbidity rates, and elevated suicide rates," diabetes, heart disease, and extreme acts of domestic violence (Bourassa & Hampton, 2004, p. 23; Brennan, 2011; Mathyssen, 2011). Perpetuation of these concerns stems from intergenerational suffering, maintaining an Indigenous identity, scepticism in colonial authorities, and feeling *othered* for racial inferiority by the host culture (Spence et al., 2016). Sources have indicated that understanding Indigenous healing practices and implementing culturally responsive and holistic care would break barriers, ameliorate treatment options for this demographic, and dismantle intergenerational cycles (Blue et al., 2015; Kirmayer et al., 2003).

Capitalism

The term "capitalism" first made its appearance in the late 1800s; Marx described it as a sociopolitical movement that valued production and influenced the modern economy (Amable, 2004). Undeniably, in current day, capitalism is based on the economic systems that emphasize commodification and the accumulation of capital. van Dijk et al. (2020) state:

The meritocratic perspective suggests that an individual's capabilities drive performance and determine the opportunities and rewards that one accumulates over time. Although this does entail that inequalities over time accumulate in workplaces, such cumulative inequalities are based on individual differences in capabilities and not based on social group membership.

(p. 243)

Capitalism causes unnecessary intersectional barriers for BIPOC, particularly in terms of the social and economic contributions that are expected of these communities. Immigrants may be inclined to identify with capitalism to prove one's professional success and achievements. There is an extra layer of guilt for immigrants, who may believe they are "never good enough" coupled with the need to "produce" and earn their stay within the host culture. This can clearly be observed within the realm of slavery and the shocking impact that the white supremacist capitalist system had on the generations of black communities (Williams, 1944; Winters, 2020). The same can be said about Indigenous communities with the *Indian Civilization Act* and having their land and resources stolen by capitalist corporations and industries (Coates, 2008; Jalata, 2011; Simon, 2011). The intersectional caste system in India during British imperialism created socioecological incongruency in the value systems held by these groups (Mosse, 2018). Noticeably, BIPOC groups have been affected by these oppressive systems, which has led to core beliefs such as unworthiness or feelings of inadequacy.

Colonialism

Modern colonialism (often used interchangeably with the term "imperialism") commenced with the Portuguese "Age of Discovery" in 1415 (Ellerkamp, 2016). Colonized lands are primarily populated, inhabited, and politically dominated by European settlers in areas such as North America, and parts of South America, Asia, Australia, and New Zealand (Glenn, 2015; Veracini, 2010). The impact of colonialism has been profound in North America for over 500 years, demonstrating a lack of respect for Indigenous culture, traditions, and territories (Gilley, 2017). As proposed by Robert Blauner (1969), creator of *Internal Colonialism*, there are four components that comprise colonization:

1. "Forced and involuntary entry" into the Indigenous land, territory, and its associated population.
2. Colonizers' effect on one's culture and patterns of social organization that strategically harm, eliminate, and/or modify Indigenous beliefs, traditions, values.
3. Power and social domination of the Indigenous population by the colonizers.
4. Racism and other forms of oppression towards the Indigenous, as a result of being viewed "inferior or different in terms of alleged biological characteristics" (p. 396).

These considerations support current economic, cultural, and language practices within these colonized lands. However, systemic racism continues to be the most damaging aspect of colonization.

Patriarchy

Patriarchy is defined as "naming gender inequality or gendered power relationships between women and men" (Patil, 2013, p. 847), which is thus used as a means of gender oppression. Some theorists believe that patriarchy originated from Charles Darwin's research, as he observed a discrepancy between the sizes of male and female statures and from that point onward, patriarchal ideologies burgeoned (Potts & Campbell, 2008, p. 171). From there, these patriarchal beliefs proliferated to include possession and control of women during courtship/marriage, domestic concerns, childbearing, and entering the labour market.

Patriarchy is fairly evident, ingrained worldwide, and is especially obvious in the mistreatment and conditioning of BIPOC women (Bourassa et al., 2004). Further sentience of this globally ingrained and archaic perspective as well as recognizing the intersectionality of women and their rights is crucial in the annihilation of the patriarchy consciousness (Patil, 2013). By fostering this awareness, men will have a better understanding of their passé and conflictual mindset, the overall impact of said mindset on feminism, and how this mindset affects the political positioning of women.

To consolidate information from chapters 4 and 5, I created the systemic oppression pyramid (see Figure 4.1) which identifies the progressive stages of how racism impacts members of a BIPOC community. This process starts at the bottom of the image with colonialism from white settlers who exploit and occupy land from Indigenous groups, spread their white supremacy and dominance, and propagate ideologies of individualism consisting of personal autonomy and independent decision-making (Tuck & Yang, 2012). White supremacy assents to the belief of being better than all other races and that white people thus have the right to dominate civilization (DiAngelo, 2011; Gillborn, 2006). These Western viewpoints support capitalism, which both divides individuals into different socioeconomic categories while patriarchal messages dictate gender and social privilege (Wills, 2018). Meritocracy suggests that we thrive in a society that honours a strong sense of professionalism and work ethic (Cech, 2013). Racial communities will then experience racial inequity in both society and occupational industries and everyday racism (e.g., microaggressions and discrimination which have now led to an increase in reported hate crimes and racial trauma). Stages of this framework

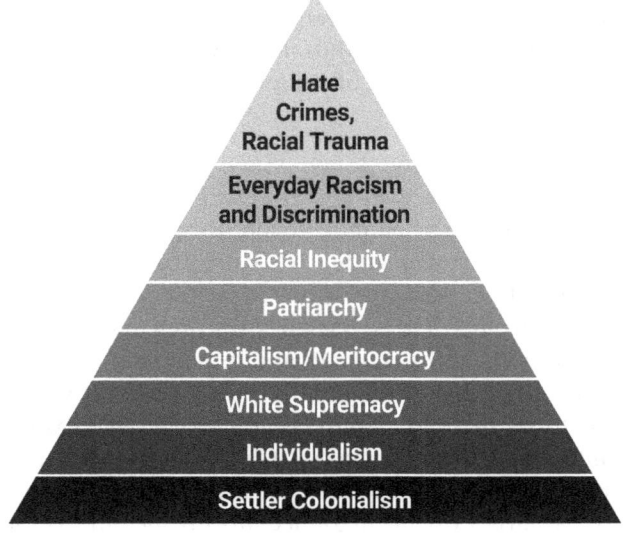

Figure 4.1 The systemic oppression pyramid

pertaining to race and what is required to combat the initial stages of racism are further reinforced in Chapter 5.

This framework is reflective of bell hooks' (2000) terminology "white supremacist capitalist patriarchy" (p. 109) to amplify power, privilege, and racial dynamics that originate with settler colonialism and their need to exert their whiteness and Western philosophies within our society. As the book progresses, we continue to learn ways of decentring these white foundations/systems of oppressions and replace them with more decolonized approaches.

References

Allan, B., & Smylie, J. (2015). *First peoples, second class treatment: The role of racism in the health and well-being of Indigenous peoples in Canada*. Wellesley Institute.

Amable, B. (2004). *The diversity of modern capitalism*. Oxford University Press.

Bell, D. (1995). Who's afraid of critical race theory? *University of Illinois Law Review, 4*, 893–910.

Bhatt, G., Tonks, R. G., & Berry, J. W. (2013). Culture in the history of psychology in Canada. *Canadian Psychology/Psychologie canadienne, 54*(2), 115–123.

Blauner, R. (1969). Internal colonialism and ghetto revolt. *Social Problems, 16*(4), 393–408.

Blue, A. W., Darou, W. G., & Ruano, C. (2015). Through silence we speak: Approaches to counselling and psychotherapy with Canadian First Nation clients. *Online Readings in Psychology and Culture, 10*(3), 3–42.

Bourassa, C., McKay-McNabb, K., & Hampton, M. (2004). Racism, sexism and colonialism: The impact on the health of Aboriginal women in Canada. *Canadian Woman Studies, 24*(1), 23–30.

Braveman, P. A., Arkin, E., Proctor, D., Kauh, T., & Holm, N. (2022). Systemic and structural racism: Definitions, examples, health damages, and approaches to dismantling. *Health Affairs, 41*(2), 171–178.

Brennan, S. (2011). *Violent victimization of Aboriginal women in the Canadian provinces, 2009*. Statistics Canada, Catalogue # 85-002-x, Juristat.

Cech, E. A. (2013). The (mis)framing of social justice: Why ideologies of depoliticization and meritocracy hinder engineers' ability to think about social injustices. In J. Lucena (Ed.), *Engineering education for social justice: Philosophy of engineering and technology* (Vol. 10, pp. 67–84). Springer Publishing Company.

Christian, M. (2019). A Global critical race and racism framework: Racial entanglements and deep and malleable whiteness. *Sociology of Race and Ethnicity, 5*(2), 169–185.

Clair, M., & Denis, J. S. (2015). Sociology of racism. In J. D. Wright (Ed.), *The international encyclopedia of the social and behavioral sciences* (Vol. 19, pp. 857–863). Elsevier.

Coates, K. (2008). The Indian Act and the future of Aboriginal governance in Canada. *National Centre for First Nations Governance*. Retrieved September 20, 2021, from www.fngovernance.org/ncfng_research/coates.pdf

Collins, P. H. (2015). Intersectionality's definitional dilemmas. *Annual Review of Sociology, 41*, 1–20.

Collins, P. H., & Bilge, S. (2016). *Intersectionality: Key concepts*. Polity Press.

Crenshaw, K. (1989). Demarginalizing the intersection of race and sex: A black feminist critique of antidiscrimination doctrine, feminist theory and antiracist politics. *University of Chicago Legal Forum, 140*, 139–167.

Crenshaw, K. (1991). Mapping the margins: Intersectionality, identity politics, and violence against women of color. *Stanford Law Review, 43*(6), 1241–1299.

Crenshaw, K. (2022). *Intersectionality: Essential writings*. The New Press.

CRIAW. (2009, June). *Everyone belongs: A toolkit for applying intersectionality*. CRIAW.

Davis, A. Y. (1983). *Women, race & class*. Vintage Books.

De La Garza, A. T., & Ono, K. A. (2016). Critical race theory. In *The international encyclopedia of communication theory and philosophy* (pp. 1–9). Wiley Blackwell.

Delgado, D., & Stefancic, J. (2017). *Critical race theory: An introduction* (3rd ed.). NYU Press.

DiAngelo, R. (2011). White fragility. *International Journal of Critical Pedagogy, 3*(3), 54–70.

DiAngelo, R. (2018). *White fragility: Why it's so hard for white people to talk about racism*. Beacon Press.

Ellerkamp, P. (2016). The first globalization: Portugal, the age of exploration, and engaging the "other" in the fifteenth and sixteenth centuries (2016). *History Theses, 22*. https://soundideas.pugetsound.edu/history_theses/22

Fonseca, S. (2020). Institutional racism in Canada: Indigenous lived realities. *The Society: Sociology and Criminology Undergraduate Review, 5*(1), 50–59.

Freire, P. (1970). *Pedagogy of the oppressed*. Continuum International.

Frieson, B. L. (2022). "It's like they don't see us at all": A critical race theory critique of dual language bilingual education for black children. *Annual Review of Applied Linguistics, 42*, 47–54.

Gee, G. C., & Ford, C. L. (2011). Structural racism and health inequities. *Du Bois Review: Social Science Research on Race, 8*(1), 115–132.

Gillborn, D. (2006). Rethinking white supremacy. *Ethnicities, 6*(3), 318–340.

Gilley, B. (2017). The case for colonialism. *Third World Quarterly*, 1–17.

Glenn, E. N. (2015). Settler colonialism as structure: A framework for comparative studies of U.S. race and gender formation. *Sociology of Race and Ethnicity, 1*(1), 52–72.

Hartlep, N. D. (2009). Critical race theory: An examination of its past, present, and future implications. *ERIC*. Retrieved July 29, 2021, from https://files.eric.ed.gov/fulltext/ED506735.pdf

Hiraldo, P. (2010). The role of critical race theory in higher education. *The Vermont Connection, 31*(1). https://scholarworks.uvm.edu/tvc/vol31/iss1/7

Hogarth, K., & Fletcher, W. L. (2018). *A space for race: Decoding racism, multiculturalism and post-colonialism and the quest for belonging in Canada and beyond*. Oxford University Press.

hooks, bell. (2000). *Feminist theory: From margin to center*. Pluto Press.

Jalata, A. (2011). Indigenous peoples in the capitalist world system: Researching, knowing, and promoting social justice. *Sociology Publications and Other Works*, 1–40.

Kirmayer, L. J., Gone, J. P., & Moses, J. (2014). Rethinking historical trauma. *Transcultural Psychiatry, 51*(3), 299–319.

Kirmayer, L. J., Simpson, C., & Cargo, M. (2003). Healing traditions: Culture, community and mental health promotion with Canadian Aboriginal peoples. *Australasian Psychiatry, 11*(1), 15–23.

Kitching, G. T., Firestone, M., Schei, B., Wolfe, S., Bourgeois, C., O'Campo, P., Rotondi, M., Nisenbaum, R., Maddox, R., & Smylie, J. (2020). Unmet health needs and discrimination by healthcare providers among an Indigenous population in Toronto, Canada. *Canadian Journal of Public Health, 111*(1), 40–49.

Lorde, A. (1992). Age, race, class, and sex: Women redefining difference. In M. Andersen & P. Hill Collins (Eds.), *Race, class, and gender: An anthology* (pp. 495–502). Wadsworth.

Marable, M. (1992). *Black America*. Open Media.

Mathyssen, I. (2011). *Ending violence against Aboriginal women and girls: Empowerment – a new beginning: Report of the standing committee on the status of women*. Standing Committee on the Status of Women.

McKague, O. (1991). *Racism in Canada*. Fifth House Publishers.

Mosse, D. (2018). Caste and development: Contemporary perspectives on a structure of discrimination and advantage. *World Development, 110*, 422–436.

Musto, R. J. (1990). Indian reserves: Canada's developing nations. *Canadian Family Physician, 36*, 105–108, 116.

Patil, V. (2013). From patriarchy to intersectionality: A transnational feminist assessment of how far we've really come. *Signs, 38*(4), 847–867.

Potts, M., & Campbell, M. (2008). The origins and future of patriarchy: The biological background of gender politics. *The Journal of Family Planning and Reproductive Healthcare, 34*(3), 171–174.

Seth, V. (2020). The origins of racism: A critique of the history of ideas. *History & Theory, 59*(3), 343–368.

Shiao, J., & Woody, A. (2021). The meaning of "racism." *Sociological Perspectives, 64*(4), 495–517.

Shramko, M., Pfluger, L., & Harrison, B. (2019). *Intersectionality and trauma-informed applications for maternal and child health research and evaluation: An initial summary of the literature*. Minnesota Department of Health.

Simon, S. (2011). Introduction: Indigenous peoples, Marxism and late capitalism. *New Proposals: Journal of Marxism and Interdisciplinary Inquiry, 5*(1), 6–9.

Solórzano, D., Allen, W., & Carroll, G. (2002). A case study of racial microaggressions and campus racial climate at the University of California, Berkeley. *UCLA Chicano/Latino Law Review, 23*, 15–111.

Spence, N. D., Wells, S., Graham, K., & George, J. (2016). Racial discrimination, cultural resilience, and stress. *The Canadian Journal of Psychiatry, 61*(5), 298–307.

Statistics Canada. (2021). *A snapshot: Status First Nations people in Canada*. Retrieved October 22, 2021, from www150.statcan.gc.ca/n1/pub/41-20-0002/412000022021001-eng.html

Steinmetz, K. (2020). She coined the term 'Intersectionality' over 30 years ago. Here's what it means to her today. *Time Magazine*. Retrieved August 10, 2022, from https://time.com/5786710/kimberle-crenshaw-intersectionality/.

Teitelbaum, K. (2022). Curriculum, conflict, and critical race theory. *Phi Delta Kappan, 103*(5), 47–53.

Tuck, E., & Yang, W. K. (2012). Decolonization is not a metaphor. *Decolonization: Indigeneity, Education & Society, 1*(1), 1–40.

van Dijk, H., Kooij, D., Karanika-Murray, M., De Vos, A., & Meyer, B. (2020). Meritocracy a myth? A multilevel perspective of how social inequality accumulates through work. *Organizational Psychology Review, 10*(3–4), 240–269.

Veracini, L. (2010). *Settler colonialism: A theoretical overview*. Palgrave MacMillan.

Viruell-Fuentes, E. A., Miranda, P. Y., & Abdulrahim, S. (2012). More than culture: Structural racism, intersectionality theory, and immigrant health. *Social Science & Medicine, 75*, 2099–2106.

Williams, E. (1944). *Capitalism and slavery*. The William Byrd Press Inc.

Wills, V. (2018). What could it mean to say, "capitalism causes sexism and racism?" *Philosophical Topics*, 46(2), 229–246.

Winters, M. F. (2020). *Black fatigue: How racism erodes the mind, body, and spirit*. Berrett-Koehler Publishers, Inc.

Chapter 5

Levels, Forms, and Movements of Racism

Building upon what is examined in Chapter 4, this chapter sheds light on the levels and forms of racism, interminority racism, racial gaslighting, internalized white supremacy, white privilege, naming one's white fragility and white guilt, latent racism, shadeism, and colourism. Additionally, Islamophobia, Sikhphobia, Black Lives Matter, and Indigenous Rights are explored.

Levels of Racism

Quite succinctly, the levels of racism include individual, systemic, everyday, and internalized racism. Each play an integral role in how racism and discrimination are perceived in distinct ecosystems, whether it be within the home, academic setting, community, or host culture (Sodhi, 2017). Each of these levels are examined below.

Individual Racism

As noted in Chapter 4, individual racism is the subjective acquisition of conscious/unconscious and personal biases and prejudice that are often influenced by one's cultural values, beliefs, and interpersonal relationships (Clair & Denis, 2015). Individual racism may take the form of internalized privilege, internalized oppression, and white supremacy. We all hold stereotypes and prejudices towards other racialized groups due to our social interactions and implicit biases.

Systemic Racism

By definition, systemic racism consists of the policies, procedures, structures, and institutes that support racial inequality and a racially oppressive system that consequently oppresses minoritized groups and people of colour (Shiao & Woody, 2021).

DOI: 10.4324/9781003216568-8

In wake of hate crimes that occurred in Atlanta and Indianapolis in April 2021, individuals were brought to a familiar place of sadness and anger over the lack of compassion towards racialized individuals. A hate crime is "a criminal offence against a person or property motivated in whole or in part by an offender's bias against a race, religion, disability, sexual orientation, ethnicity, gender or gender identity" (American Psychological Association, 2021).

To help process these incomprehensible hate crimes, BIPOC and white individuals alike can reframe their perspective and contribute as a productive ally, in hopes that there will be a better understanding around systemic racism and the clout it has on our global society. Steps towards eliminating systemic racism are as follows:

- Sit with discomfort and lack of awareness about racism.
- Listen and unlearn; acknowledge the trajectory required to understand racism.
- Implement privilege in an effective manner.
- Influence others to become culturally responsive and respectful.
- Discuss current topics about racism at home and in academic settings, and within the community and host culture.
- Continue the dialogue about racism; engage in constructive communication about these matters.

Everyday Racism

According to Philomena Essed (1991):

> Everyday racism has been defined as the process in which socialized racist notions are integrated into everyday practices and thereby actualize and reinforce underlying racial and ethnic relations. Furthermore, racist practices in themselves become familiar, repetitive, and part of the "normal" routine in everyday life.
>
> (p. 145)

While we live in white dominated societies, acts associated with everyday racism continue to immobilize BIPOC communities regardless of the context. Whether a person is a target of a premeditated hate crime or police brutality, posting on social media platforms is not enough to amplify and end racial injustice. Collective humanity needs to speak more about sustainable anti-racist practices. Until these initiatives are implemented, BIPOC will endure "the psychological distress due to racism on a day-to-day basis which can have chronic adverse effects on their mental and physical health" (Essed, 1991).

Types of everyday racism are microaggressions, negative assumptions of intellectual inferiority towards a cultural/ethnic/racial demographic, endorsement of the model minority myth, racial denigration, ignorance about racism, racist humour, ethnic jokes, hate crimes, police brutality, criminalization of a racial group, and reluctance to become a productive anti-racist ally.

BIPOC are commonly targeted with everyday racism; a particularly frequent issue, especially for Asian and South Asian individuals (Shams, 2020) are stereotypes regarding the model minority myth. Yi et al. (2020) state, "The myth is often defined as the overgeneralization that Asian Americans achieve universal educational and occupational success" (p. 543). This myth is being supplanted, but unfortunately by anti-Asian racism associated with the COVID-19 pandemic. This anti-Asian hatred has elevated fear, the number of hate crime and discriminatory incidents, and racial injustice as this population receives harsh microaggressions alongside blame for causing the COVID-19 pandemic (Choi, 2021; Kim, 1999).

The model minority myth perception was created during the 1800s but flourished during the mid-twentieth century as Asians immigrated to North America. A key component of this myth were and are comparisons between Asian and black work ethic (Yi & Museus, 2015). Such differentiations may provide Asians job security and sense of belonging in the Western culture and labour market; yet to this day, expectations regarding immigrant performance and contribution to the Western capitalist economy persist (Shams, 2020). Stereotypes related to the model minority myth yield consequences such as cultural dissonance, colour blindness (failure to recognize race), and a lack of acknowledgement about the barriers that Asians experience. Additional stereotypes are the misconception that Asians have no tribulations and can do no wrong, as well as the awkward social positioning of Asians who are perceived as "better" than other racial groups (Matsuda, 1990; Museus, 2013).

The model minority myth can have severe mental health consequences for Asians (Gupta et al., 2011; Viruell-Fuentes, 2012). A 2018 study conducted by Noh (2018) examined how the role of the model minority myth specifically influences the suicidality of Asian American women. The findings suggest that this form of everyday racism causes unwarranted internalized stress whereby individuals feel blamed for not meeting societal expectations; she calls for further awareness and resources to assist this demographic.

The term *microaggression* was first coined in the 1960s by Dr. Chester Pierce, an African American psychiatrist, to describe the "subtle, stunning, often automatic, and non-verbal exchanges which are 'put downs'" (Pierce et al., 1978, p. 66). Expanding on this definition, Sue et al. (2007) convey that microaggressions are "brief and commonplace daily verbal, behavioural, and environmental indignities, whether intentional or unintentional, that communicate hostile, derogatory, or negative racial slights and insults to the target person or group" (p. 273). As such, racial microaggressions can fall under three themes: microassaults, microinsults, and microinvalidations (Sue et al., 2007).

1. **Microassaults** are intentional and defamatory comments or name calling that are specific to the individual's racial or cultural identity (e.g., referring to someone as "coloured," calling them a racial label, or making a racist joke).
2. **Microinsults** are seemingly unintentional comments or questions that demonstrate insensitivity and lack of respect to an individual's ethnic, cultural, or racial background (e.g., questioning one's qualifications due to race or ethnicity).
3. **Microinvalidations** dismiss a BIPOC's thoughts, feelings, sentiments, and hardship (e.g., colour blindness or commenting on how racism is not real).

These themes reinforce the everyday hardships experienced by BIPOC and their need to resort to internalized racism.

> *Some examples of microaggressions are: "Where are you really from?", "You speak good English for an immigrant!", "You're so whitewashed!", "Why do people of your community . . . ?", and "Your people are taking all of OUR jobs!"*

Microaggressions are a modern form of racism that are obvious and deliberate due to past historical or racial concerns; however, microaggressions can be covert and draining. Microaggressions can compound internalized racism and thus lead to mistrust in Western culture, no sense of belonging, and mental health concerns such as heightened anxiety or depression (Cénat et al., 2021; Houshmand et al., 2017; Sodhi, 2017).

Internalized Racism

Internalized racism or internalized white supremacy infers "the individual inculcation of the racist stereotypes, values, images, and ideologies perpetuated by the white dominant society about one's racial group, leading to feelings of self-doubt, disgust, and disrespect for one's race and/or oneself" (Pyke, 2010, p. 553). Internalized racism results from racial gaslighting, tone policing, and microaggressions, which are discussed in this chapter. Within my clinical practice, I have explored whether internalized racism is a part of an immigrant's acculturation process and/or a defence mechanism to preclude feeling othered by members of the host country. Is it just easier to identify with the host country? Is this the only option?

There is a plethora of reasons why racism contributes to immigrants and BIPOC feeling victimized, thereby succumbing to internalized racism: feeling incongruent and lacking belongingness in either culture; encountering indifference and possibly resentment towards their ancestral culture from within themselves; being subjugated and powerless; and experiencing fear and ambiguity upon encountering racial microaggressions and discrimination (David et al., 2019). Here is a personal example of how I reframed and unlearned internalized racism:

> Upon moving to Nova Scotia, my parents decided that English would become our first language, instead of Punjabi. They believed that by speaking English, we would have an easier time "fitting in" with our Canadian peers and Nova Scotian culture. My grandparents felt the same way when the British colonized India, or perhaps learning English was considered a status symbol of sorts. Reflecting upon this language choice, I recognize specific forms of internalized racism: proximity privilege to the host culture, people pleasing, and shedding a part of our collective cultural identity. From the age of eight, I chose to resolve this by reclaiming my language and decided to teach myself Punjabi and have encouraged my daughters to do the same.

I learned to heal from internalized racism and empower my clients to do the same by:

- Nurturing a positive racial and/or ethnic identity.
- Unlearning racial stereotypes and biases.
- Addressing visceral responses to racial microaggressions.
- Navigating covert/latent and overt racism.
- Developing an assertive and resilient disposition.
- Becoming a productive anti-racist ally.
- Engaging in purposeful dialogue about racism.
- Educating others about the impact of racism on BIPOC communities.

Mending the wounds of internalized racism can begin anywhere, and doing so on an individual level may translate to systemic change.

Is normalizing racism essentially internalizing racism? To what extent do we surrender to the patriarchal white supremist oppressive systems? Figure 5.1 illustrates the overlap between normalizing racism and toxic positivity.

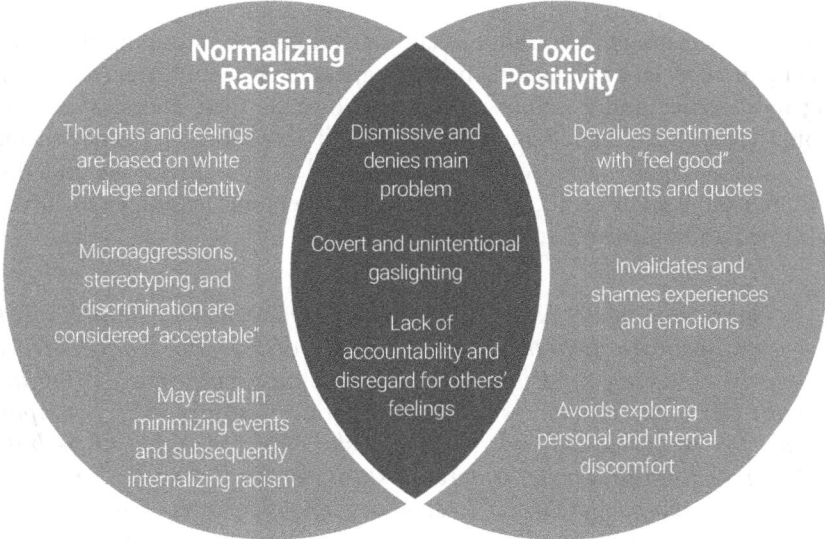

Figure 5.1 Normalizing racism versus toxic positivity

At the heart of this diagram is the idea that prioritizing the emotional needs and feelings of others over our own hinders personal and authentic growth for all involved. Therapy or psychoeducation for BIPOC clients who grapple with the effects of normalized racism may involve examining the precursors (e.g., undiagnosed mental health conditions, unresolved trauma, inner child wounds, or attachment concerns discussed in Chapter 3) for the beliefs highlighted in the image.

Forms of Racism

Interminority Racism

Interminority racism refers to the prejudice, discrimination, and power imbalances that occur between racial and ethnic groups. This form of racism is becoming increasingly universal but is not well documented due to its controversial nature (Harbi, 2016; Lee et al., 2019; Natapoff, 1995; Singh, 2019). Bivens (2005) explains that:

> Internalized racism negatively impacts people of color intra-culturally and cross-culturally. Because race is a social and political construct that comes out of histories of domination and exploitation between Peoples, people of colors' internalized racism often led to great conflict among and between them as other concepts of power – such as ethnicity, culture, nationality and class – are collapsed in misunderstanding.
>
> (p. 45)

Even within a culture or communities, one can observe forms of discrimination based on skin colour, such as shadeism and colourism. There have been conflicting social insinuations and references made about the benefits of being fair complexioned, which again brings a person to closer proximity to whiteness (proximity privilege). Darker-skinned people appear to be most oppressed, as noted on this white-black continuum:

> *My eldest daughter has been treated differently throughout her lifetime due to her skin colour. For example, when employed at a long-term care facility, she would return home and relay occurrences of everyday racism committed by her coworkers and residents of the home alike. She referenced these experiences when talking about how self-conscious she feels about her skin colour and how it is represented here in Canada. My younger daughter has fairer skin, has not experienced any form of racism, and appears more comfortable "in her skin" than my eldest daughter.*

Inherent within interminority racism is a dichotomy of sorts; we honour Asian individuals for their strong work ethic rooted within the minority model myth, yet we are simultaneously endorsing anti-Asian racism and blaming Asians for the cause of the COVID-19 pandemic (Choi, 2021). This continues to be true of other cultural and racial groups. To be both the "chosen" ones and to be mistreated and shunned by other cultural groups is a common feature of interminority racism.

Islamophobia and Sikhphobia

Islamophobia is anti-Muslim racism. It commenced during the religious and political rivalries within Egypt, Damascus, and Jerusalem during the twentieth century (Bakali, 2016). This inevitably resulted in fearing the Islam democracy due to their threatening disposition towards the Church of Western Europe, primarily comprised of the Roman Catholic Church. Bakali (2016) articulates, "Postcolonial theorists have examined the impacts of colonialism on both the colonized and colonizers, who have benefited from the violence and promotion of racist ideology resulting from colonization" (p. 12). This passage emphasizes the importance of decentring Islamophobia:

> *During the summer of 2022, my daughters and I watched Ms. Marvel, a series that highlighted a South Asian teen superhero. Each episode essentially demystified Islamophobia; watching this series with my daughters was empowering. They learned about the Muslim community, Pakistani wedding ceremonies, and the 1947 Partition of India/Pakistan. We also understood the Urdu language due to similarities between Urdu and Punjabi. Both daughters commented on how there should be more Marvel characters with South Asian backgrounds, as representation combats racism and teaches mainstream culture about our collective culture, history, and language.*

The dissemination of Islamophobia is based on colonized views and mindsets that assume all Muslims are terrorists and a threat to Western civilization, as we have seen post-9/11 with Al-Qaeda, (Al-Solaylee, 2016; Sidhu, 2013). As I write this section of the book, it is mere days before the 20th anniversary of 9/11. With this monumental anniversary on the horizon, will there be further retaliation towards Muslim people? This form of discrimination, unfortunately, extended to other cultures who resembled Muslims. Racists are not known to be nuanced and are unable to differentiate between cultural groups; for example, Muslims and Sikhs are the same group to racists (Ahluwalia & Pellettiere, 2010; O'Donnell et al., 2018). Sharing similar stereotypical physical characteristics, namely darker skin, beards, and turbans, Sikh males have often been erroneously assumed for Muslim males and have been mistakenly targeted as a result (Shams, 2020; Sidhu, 2013). Western culture conflates Muslims for Sikhs and vice versa.

Sikhphobia, a subconstruct of xenophobia, is an anti-Sikh sentiment that is derived from the prejudice, demonization, and discrimination against individuals from different cultural and/or religious backgrounds (Ahluwalia & Pellettiere, 2010; Awan, 2010). The genesis of Sikhphobia burgeoned from 1947 Partition of India/Pakistan and further reinforced in the 1980s during Indira Gandhi's term as prime minister of India (Gautam, 2021). As the importance of unlearning Islamophobia, Sikhphobia, and xenophobia continues to be debated, the merging of the two religious groups is apparent in hate crimes that are specifically directed towards Muslim individuals (Birk et al., 2015).

Racism and trauma can occur simultaneously and repeatedly in the form of hate crimes. Racist acts of violence are rising and being reported worldwide due to social and globalized media. Perhaps hate crimes have existed without a name over the last century. Hate crimes have become more prevalent around the globe since 9/11, in bigger urban centres but equally in small North American towns. Not all hate crimes make it to national or international news or even social media outlets, nor do they gain remarkable media coverage. As a collective global community, are we enabling these Islamophobic violent events from happening? For over 20 years, since 9/11, there has been an increase in wrongfully targeted hate crime against Muslim, black, and brown communities within North America. The first reported incident occurred on September 15, 2001, towards a Sikh man, Balbir Singh Sodhi (no relation), who resided in Arizona (Kaur, 2021). He was killed because he was believed to be Muslim due to his turban and beard. Several South Asian hate crimes followed; racists attacked individuals with a stereotypical Muslim appearance and/or "racialized otherness" (Shams, 2020). Whether these were premeditated individualized attacks or in a *Mosque* (an Islamic place of worship) or *Gurdwara* (Sikh temple), as in the 2012 Oak Creek shooting, confusion around discerning between Muslims and Sikhs continues to take place with very little change or awareness in sight (Birk et al., 2015; Kaur, 2021).

Hate crimes since 2020 fuelled by colonial and white supremacist ignorance include the following: police brutality involving George Floyd, the Atlanta anti-Asian shooting, and the Indianapolis anti-Sikh shooting. There are probably more that have not been reported. One event literally hit close to my hometown, Halifax, six days before the twentieth anniversary of 9/11. In the rural town of Truro, Nova Scotia, a 23-year-old Sikh man was murdered for no apparent reason. He was returning home from work when he was attacked and killed outside of his apartment. This is a suspected hate crime as no robbery was committed. He migrated from Punjab, India, to Canada in 2017 as an international student and was working two jobs to support his family in India. This event shocked the Nova Scotian Sikh community; many felt extremely vulnerable and unsafe while collectively contending with this trauma. There was minimal media coverage and reporting about this hate crime within North America. Are hate crimes becoming normalized? Again, when will immigrants and BIPOC matter? How are they going to feel safe in their *pardes* or adopted homeland?

Racial Gaslighting

The term gaslighting originates from the 1944 movie titled *Gaslight* in which the main character manipulates and controls his spouse by turning down a gas lantern and telling her she is imagining that he is doing so (Tobias & Joseph, 2020). Fast forward to the twenty-first century, and particularly with the undercurrents of white supremacy within North America, racial gaslighting is alive and well. Racial gaslighting, a form of manipulation and psychological abuse, can be defined as "the political, social, economic and cultural process that perpetuates and normalizes a white supremacist reality through pathologizing those who resist" (Davis & Ernst, 2019, p. 761).

Inspired by the work of Roberts and Andrews (2013, p. 78), Tobias and Joseph (2020, p. 233) discuss five aspects of the gaslighting process:

1. The gaslighter is a person or group who manipulates reality because they can benefit from doing so.
2. The gaslightee is the person/persons whose reality/lived experience are manipulated and distorted by the gaslighter. Usually, the gaslightee represents either figurative or literal reward for the gaslighter.
3. The third component is the object of manipulation. The object of manipulation is usually the persons, events, or objects that the gaslighter manipulates to distort and alter the gaslightee's memory.
4. The fourth component of gaslighting is the consequence(s) experienced by the gaslightee. The consequence(s) experienced by the gaslightee are detrimental and can impact them financially, socially, mentally, physically, and emotionally.
5. The fifth component of gaslighting is the reward(s) for the gaslighter. The reward(s) for the gaslighter can be described through two parts: the results of the gaslighter's actions and the advantage that the gaslighter receives over the gaslightee as a result of the gaslighting.

An example of racial gaslighting is *tone policing*, in which individuals further oppress and patronize the tone and communication style of marginalized community members. Other examples may be: *"Racism doesn't exist anymore." "I don't see colour," "Why is it always about race?", "I was only joking, calm down!", "You're being too sensitive," and "What I said wasn't racist."* The privileged individual dismisses the emotion of the oppressed individual's statement.

White Privilege

White privilege involves the numerous opportunities available to those individuals who identify as *white* or *white passing*. White individuals are supported in a position of power and contribute to an "institution predominantly operated *by* white people *for* white people" (Gillborn, 2006, p. 319). Even with this power and authority over other, this privilege is rarely used to combat racism, capitalism, or diminish white supremist hate crimes towards others (Bhopal, 2018; Carr, 2016).

There is a clear intersection between white privilege and white supremacy. Due to their race, white individuals have advantages and superiority within the dominant culture over other racial and cultural groups. I am reminded of the wise words of hooks and Mesa-Bains (2006): "privilege is not in and of itself bad; what matters is what we do with privilege. Privilege does not have to be negative, but we must share our resources and take direction about how to use our privilege in ways that empower those who lack it" (p. 76). In the opinion of Sojonky (2010), "white privilege refers to a system of advantages, benefits and opportunities experienced by white persons in our society simply by virtue of the colour of their skin" (p. 26). Blue et al. (2015) adds, "it privileges the white person educationally, economically, as well as occupationally, in terms of healthcare, housing, child-rearing, and in their reactions with various social systems" (p. 11).

White Fragility

White fragility, as explained by DiAngelo (2011), is a state that excludes white persons from acknowledging their privilege and their role in reproducing racism in the fabric of society, where "even a minimum of racial stress becomes intolerable, triggering a range of defensive moves . . . silence, anger, guilt" (p. 57). Simply said, white fragility entails the discomfort white people encounter regarding any form of social and/or racial inequality. In addition to the previously noted emotions, other responses might include silence, fear, shame, denial, insecurity, and disagreement. Unresolved emotions may create various forms of barriers that prevent white people from adequately discussing racism with marginalized members of society. These emotions moreover hinder white people from contending with their internalized white guilt, which is "the degree to which feeling remorseful about racism and racial inequality may facilitate or inhibit antiracist attitudes and behavior" (Grzanka et al., 2020, p. 49).

The White Racial Affect Scale (WRAS), as mentioned in a study by Grzanka et al. (2020) measures white guilt and shame that is associated with detachment and blame. The scale is composed of the following subscales: racial argument, white guilt, psychosocial costs of racism to whites, and tests of self-conscious affect. Results of the study highlighted variations of white guilt, shame, and negation, and Grzanka et al. (2020) call for the further development of scales that examine anti-racist and racial prejudice feelings.

Due to racial privileges, white people may feel entitled to disengage or become antagonistic about racial discourse. The point here is to recognize that manifestations of white fragility (i.e., thoughts and behaviours) perpetuate racism, and that white people need to discuss the emotions they harbour that solidify this mindset. By developing "racial stamina," white people learn how to overcome racial barriers and understand the necessity to intentionally dialogue about racism with BIPOC (DiAngelo, 2018; Grzanka et al., 2020). Racial stamina is not synonymous with being "woke." Instead, racial stamina encourages white people to consider their positions of power and privilege, internalized racial biases and consciousness, and the urgency to have intentional conversations about racism with BIPOC.

Racial stamina involves consistently and intentionally showing up for BIPOC and becoming more engaged in the productive allyship ventures (Akbar, 2020). A progression of sorts might start with reading and/or attending trainings on cultural responsiveness and/or reading a book about anti-racism, then raising awareness about *Black Lives Matter*, and finally demonstrating endurance by participating in community-led solidarity vigil in honour of hate crime victims. The possibilities are endless; however, every action should be championed in an authentic and purposeful manner.

The final section of this chapter discusses movements that are supported by enduring productive allyship.

Social Justice Movements

On August 1, 2022, during a dinner time conversation with extended family, we landed on the topic of the absence of movements for Asian and other marginalized groups. Even though these concerns are being further magnified, there are very few exclusive social justice campaigns for Asian, South Asian, and Latine groups (e.g., "Stop Asian Hate"). Throughout this book, I outline BIPOC communities and the diverse oppressions they have suffered. However, to punctuate the end of this chapter, there is a discussion of two highly profiled movements: *Black Lives Matter* and *Indigenous Rights*.

Black Lives Matter

Black history in North America is extensive. The first black individual set foot on North American soil in the early 1500s, and the first documented enslaved Africans arrived on colonized land in 1619. This was the start of forced migration to Canada and the United States from either the Caribbean or Africa due to enslavement (Statistics Canada, 2019). Conventional hegemonic ideals prevailed as the colonizers assumed the roles of masters and the displaced Africans as their slaves. The command by virtue of power and position was evident over the years, and particularly through dominant culture privilege.

Black communities have been stereotyped as people who are criminals and social misfits since enslavement. As the following passages indicate, these stereotypes are clearly embedded in colonial and racial domination (Davis, 1983). The black community has endured significant systemic oppression and barriers that persist today (Winters, 2020). Black lives do matter, and it is not just a movement or an event that is celebrated every February; it is a lived reality for this historic demographic. What follows is written within Canadian and American contexts.

Monumental events such as the *American Revolution* (1776–1783) and the *American Civil War* (1861) emancipated slaves from colonialists which started the abolishment of slavery through the passing of the *Thirteenth Amendment to the United States Constitution* in 1865 (Blumrosen et al., 2006; Degruy, 2017). Prior to this amendment, black men, women, and children worked in cotton and sugar plantations as indentured servants. Their lifestyle consisted of working 14–18 hours, living in crowded shacks or huts, and sleeping 4–6 hours a night. The treatment that existed on these plantations has been documented as abiding to their master's commands and being punished for demonstrating any form of resistance. Disobedience resulted in abhorrent forms of physical and mental violence such as beatings and starvation.

In 1784, racial tension occurred between black slaves who were recruited by the British to fight in the American Revolution; for their service, they would receive land in Canada. Ten days of riots and conflict arose between the black loyalists and white communities in Nova Scotia when a black preacher's house was raided. Between 1815 and 1860, enslaved individuals travelled the *Underground Railroad* to migrate to Canadian provinces such as Ontario (Bakan, 2008). Unfortunately, the *Fugitive Slave Law* in 1850 emphasized the capturing of black individuals who were fleeing American states. Harriett Tubman, a former slave, is renowned for assisting others to use this railway system and eventually become liberated.

In Canada, slavery came to a halt in 1834 in part due to codes from the British *Slavery Abolition Act* (1833), although black people still experienced severe forms of racial inequality, segregation in several provincial schools (Cheboud & France, 2021; Maynard, 2017), and discrimination. The creation of enclaves such as *Africville* in Halifax, Nova Scotia, and *Hogan's Alley* in Vancouver, British Columbia, are relics of this "progress." Africville was established in the 1800s, whereas *Hogan's Alley* originated between 1915 and 1917. Both settlements were demolished in the 1960s due to racist connotations.

During the 1900s, anti-black racism incidents overlapped with political efforts to abolish racial segregation and discrimination against black citizens within America. Examples of these anti-racist efforts include the *Civil Rights Movement* (1954–1968) and the *Montgomery Bus Boycott* (1955–1956). Dr. Martin Luther King Jr., a minister, led the charge towards equality for black people with the intentions of creating federal legislation based on economic, political, and social rights for the black community. This non-violent movement contributed to protests, boycotts, marches, and sit-ins in colleges and black churches, exemplifying the importance and need for equality and freedom (Oates, 2013). The *Civil Rights Movement* culminated with the passing and implementation of a law that permitted black individuals to attend restaurants, workplaces, and schools and to use public transportation alongside white citizens.

Dr. Martin Luther King Jr. persevered to mobilize the cause to end segregation and racial inequality, particularly in his renowned 1963 speech, *I Have a Dream*, until his assassination in April 1968. His death led to further race riots in cities across the United States of America as citizens tried to make sense of this loss. Speeches by Robert F. Kennedy and others were made to quell these riots and caution any form of police brutality. To curtail racial tension, *The Civil Rights Act* of 1968 was signed into law by Lyndon B. Johnson (Massey, 2015).

During the twentieth century, there was an outstanding number of exceptional black representation: Malcolm X, Rosa Parks, James Baldwin, Audrey Lorde, Mohammed Ali, bell hooks, Maya Angelou, and Viola Davies. The twenty-first century has seen Toni Morrison, Jesse Jackson, Oprah Winfrey, Barack Obama, and other political, athletic, academic, musical, and Hollywood figures who continue to break racial barriers. Despite all this representation, still societal generalizations, intergenerational trauma, and years of systemic oppression continue to impact the black community (Davis, 1983; DeGruy, 2017).

Black Heritage Month was founded in 1915 to commemorate the 50th anniversary of emancipation from slavery. Black Heritage/History Month was first recognized in 1926 as *Negro History Week* in the United States by famous activist Carter G. Woodson, also known as the *Father of Black History* (Dagbovie, 2003). The month of February was chosen to honour both Abraham Lincoln and Fredrick Douglass, whose birthdays were in February and who significantly helped the black community. Black Heritage/History Month was first officiated in 1976 in America and 1995 in Canada. This month-long event celebrates the contributions and accomplishments made by black individuals (Landa, 2012).

Even with this annual recognition of black excellence and liberation, acrimony persists towards black members in the form of racial profiling, anti-black racism incidents, shooting innocent victims (e.g., Breonna Taylor), and police brutality (Wilkerson, 2020). Thus, the social movement *Black Lives Matter* was initiated in 2013 to overturn anti-black racism and racial inequality:

The *Black Lives Matter* movement, for instance, is now challenging the implicit caste system across North America by focussing on police brutality and how it reflects a deeper problem: historically engrained systems of racism in Canada and the United States that seep into laws and regulations as well as public and private attitudes and practices. The only answer is having all the ethnic groups work together to create an equitable society for everyone.

(Cheboud & France, 2021, p. 388)

In 1865, *Juneteenth*, a holiday to memorialize the culmination of slavery was created. Originally called *Jubilee Day*, it is celebrated annually on June 19th. Additionally, *Emancipation Day* takes place on August 1 throughout Canada, the United States, and the Caribbean. While these holidays exist, they are hardly being observed. Racial tension continues to transpire, regardless of the efforts to acknowledge and address hardships encountered by the black community (Winters, 2020). Efforts are being made to educate individuals in academia and workplaces about dismantling anti-black racism (Genao & Mercedes, 2021; Munroe, 2021). This will require all members of society to re-evaluate their privileges and oppressions and become productive allies, which is deliberated upon in Chapter 6.

Indigenous Rights

There is a dark and oppressive part of North America's history, a hidden genocide that lasted for over 125 years in Canadian (Turtle Island) Indian Residential Schools and American Indian Boarding Schools, which were comparable in the treatment and abuse towards Indigenous children (Restoule, 2013). Mandated by the *Indian Civilization Act* in Canada and supported by the Churches, it is hard to fathom the power colonization has had on one specific group. American boarding schools existed from 1819 to the 1960s, with the sole purpose of assimilating Native people into the American culture. This book focuses on the Canadian Indigenous Residential School System.

There has been tremendous dialogue about the institutional racism and tragic injustices faced by the Indigenous (First Nations, Métis, and Inuit Peoples) communities. This racism began during the inception of imperialist colonization and subsequent white supremist interventions. Several years later, the Indigenous community are mourning not only the loss of their stolen land, but lost identity and younger generations who died in residential schools (MacDonald & Hudson, 2012).

The *Indian Civilization Act* was signed into effect in 1876. In 1884, the legislation was amended to endorse the removal of Indigenous children from their families and communities due to assumptions of improper care and lack of education (Bhatt et al., 2013). These children (ages 4–16) were placed in residential schools, which were established and funded in the late 1870s by the Canadian government's Department of Indian Affairs and organized by church and religious orders. By 1920, it became mandatory for Indigenous children to attend residential schools, and approximately 150,000 First Nations, Métis, and Inuit children were enrolled. A total of approximately 139 residential schools, affiliated with the Indian Residential School System existed between the 1870s and 1996 when the last school finally closed in Saskatchewan.

In Canada, over 7,310 unmarked and mass graves were uncovered in 2021 alone, and the investigation has just begun; this is not the final count. This only covers the bodies that were found as opposed to locating individual graves. Children died of genocidal government procedures of assimilation by being separated from their families and told to abandon their culture and native languages to attend residential boarding schools throughout Canada (MacDonald & Hudson, 2012). Those who survived the multitude of hardships while attending these schools suffered from immense grief and intergenerational trauma.

These schools were created to force Indigenous children to become more Westernized, change their physical appearance (cut their braids) to look more "civilized," convert to Christianity, and assimilate into Canadian society (Fonseca, 2020). Their names were replaced with numbers. They were also verbally abused, emotionally neglected, starved, tortured, beaten, and raped. They were required to abandon their spiritual beliefs, ancestral languages, and speak English and French. As well, Elders, known for keeping the community knowledge and preserving Indigenous language, were disrespected.

Originally called *Indian Day* by Jules Sioui, *Canada National Indigenous Peoples Day* was established in 1982. It is celebrated in Canada on June 21st and affords citizens an opportunity to appreciate the histories and culture of the First Nations, Métis, and Inuit peoples. Complementing this acknowledgement, on September 30, 2021, Canada observed its first *National Day for Truth and Reconciliation*, where the legacy of First Nations, Métis, and Inuit residential school survivors and those children who did not return home, their families, and communities were honoured. With further awareness, compassion, and empathy, one could only hope that the Indigenous community will receive the support, love, and respect they ultimately deserve.

Indigenous relations issues are deeper than colonization practices of residential schools. In 2015, the *Truth and Reconciliation Report* was published (Commission of Canada, 2015) to assist Indigenous peoples in reclaiming their familial, cultural, and spiritual identities. It details the history, legacy, and challenge of reconciliation, and includes "94 Calls to Action" in the following categories: Legacy, Education, Language and Culture, Health, and Justice. The report also discusses "Reconciliation and Canadian Governments and the United Nations Declaration on the

Rights of Indigenous People" (Commission of Canada, 2015, p. 325). These initiatives were to be completed within a five-year timeframe. Further "Calls to Action" within the *Truth and Reconciliation Report* include requesting land sovereignty, improved housing conditions, clean water on reserves, and re-evaluation of the legal repercussions of Indigenous peoples (Butler et al., 2015; Restoule, 2013; Simeon, 2010; Statistics Canada, 2021).

Chapter 6 connects constructs from Chapters 4 and 5, imparts mental health implications of racism, addresses strategies to heal and become resilient, and demonstrates how to develop an anti-racist stance.

References

Ahluwalia, M. K., & Pellettiere, L. (2010). Sikh men post-9/11: Misidentification, discrimination, and coping. *Asian American Journal of Psychology, 1*(4), 303–314.

Akbar, M. (2020). *Beyond ally: The pursuit to racial justice.* Publish Your Purpose Press.

Al-Solaylee, K. (2016). *Brown: What being brown in the world today means (to everyone).* Harper Collins.

American Psychological Association. (2021). *The psychology of hate crimes.* Retrieved August 25, 2021, from www.apa.org/advocacy/interpersonal-violence/hate-crimes

Awan, M. (2010). Global terror and the rise of Xenophobia/Islamophobia: An analysis of American cultural production since September 11. *Islamic Studies, 49*(4), 521–537.

Bakali, N. (2016). Historicizing and theorizing Islamophobia and anti-Muslim racism. In *Islamophobia: Understanding anti-Muslim racism through the lived experiences of Muslim youth* (pp. 11–25). Brill.

Bakan, A. B. (2008). Reconsidering the underground railroad: Slavery and racialization in the making of the Canadian state. *Socialist Studies, 4,* 3–29.

Bhatt, G., Tonks, R. G., & Berry, J. W. (2013). Culture in the history of psychology in Canada. *Canadian Psychology, 54*(2), 115–123.

Bhopal, K. (2018). *White privilege: The myth of a post-racial society.* Policy Press.

Birk, M., Gill, H., & Heer, K. (2015). De-Islamizing Sikhphobia: Deconstructing structural racism in Wisconsin gurdwara shooting 10/12. *Education, Citizenship and Social Justice, 10,* 97–106.

Bivens, D. K. (2005). What is internalized racism? In M. Potapchuk, S. Leiderman, D. Bivens & B. Major (Eds.), *Flipping the script: White privilege and community building* (pp. 43–51). Center for Assessment and Policy Development.

Blue, A. W., Darou, W. G., & Ruano, C. (2015). Through silence we speak: Approaches to counselling and psychotherapy with Canadian First Nation clients. *Online Readings in Psychology and Culture, 10*(3), 3–42.

Blumrosen, A. W., Blumrosen, R. G., & Blumrosen, S. (2006). *Slave nation: How slavery united the colonies and sparked the American Revolution.* Sourcebooks.

Butler, J., Ng-A-Fook, N., Vaudrin-Charette, J., & McFadden, F. (2015). Living between truth and reconciliation: Responsibilities, colonial institutions, and settler scholars. *Transnational Curriculum Inquiry, 12*(2), 44–64.

Carr, P. R. (2016). Whiteness and white privilege: Problematizing race and racism in a "color-blind" world, and in education. *International Journal of Critical Pedagogy, 7*(1), 51–74.

Cénat, J. M., Hajizadeh, S., Dalexis, R. D., Ndengeyingoma, A., Guerrier, M., & Kogan, C. (2021). Prevalence and effects of daily and major experiences of racial discrimination and microaggressions among black individuals in Canada. *Journal of Interpersonal Violence, 37*(17–18), NP16750–NP16778.

Cheboud, E., & France, M. H. (2021). Counselling black Canadians. In M. H. France, M. del Carmen Rodriguez & G. G. Hett (Eds.), *Diversity, culture and counselling: A Canadian perspective* (3rd ed., pp. 276–300). Edmonton, AB: Brush Education Inc.

Choi, S. (2021). "People look at me like I am the virus": Fear, stigma, and discrimination during the COVID-19 pandemic. *Qualitative Social Work, 20*(1–2), 233–239.

Clair, M., & Denis, J. S. (2015). Sociology of racism. In J. D. Wright (Ed.), *The international encyclopedia of the social and behavioral sciences* (Vol. 19, pp. 857–863). Elsevier.

Commission of Canada. (2015). *Honouring the truth, reconciling the future, summary of the truth and reconciliation.* Commission of Canada.

Dagbovie, P. (2003). Making black history practical and popular: Carter G. Woodson, the Proto black Studies Movement and the struggle for black liberation. *Western Journal of Black Studies, 27*(4), 263–274.

David, E. J. R., Schroeder, T. M., & Fernandez, J. (2019). Internalized racism: A systematic review of the psychological literature on racism's most insidious consequence. *Journal of Social Issues, 75*(4), 1057–1086.

Davis, A. M., & Ernst, R. (2019). Racial gaslighting. *Politics, Groups, and Identities, 7*(4), 761–774.

Davis, A. Y. (1983). *Women, race & class.* Vintage Books.

Degruy, J. A. (2017). *Post traumatic slave syndrome: America's legacy of enduring injury and healing.* Joy Degruy Publications Inc.

DiAngelo, R. (2011). White fragility. *International Journal of Critical Pedagogy, 3*(3), 54–70.

DiAngelo, R. (2018). *White fragility: Why it's so hard for white people to talk about racism.* Beacon Press.

Essed, P. (1991). *Understanding everyday racism: An interdisciplinary theory.* Sage Publications.

Fonseca, S. (2020). Institutional racism in Canada: Indigenous lived realities. *The Society: Sociology and Criminology Undergraduate Review, 5*(1), 50–59.

Gautam, D. P. (2021). Affirmations of humanity amidst violence: A study of select partition stories. *Research Journal of English Language and Literature (RJELAL), 9*(2), 139–147.

Genao, S., & Mercedes, Y. (2021). All we need is one mic: A call for anti-racist solidarity to deconstruct anti-black racism in educational leadership. *Journal of School Leadership, 31*(1–2), 127–141.

Gillborn, D. (2006). Rethinking white supremacy. *Ethnicities, 6*(3), 318–340.

Grzanka, P. R., Frantell, K. A., & Fassinger, R. E. (2020). The white racial affect scale (WRAS): A measure of white guilt, shame, and negation. *The Counseling Psychologist, 48*(1), 47–77.

Gupta, A., Szymanski, D., & Leong, F. (2011). The "model minority myth": Internalized racialism of positive stereotypes as correlates of psychological distress, and attitudes toward help-seeking. *Asian American Journal of Psychology, 2*, 101–114.

Harbi, N. (2016). Inter-minority racial prejudice and anti-white bias: An underestimated phenomenon. *Expressions, 1*(2), 138–147.

hooks, b., & Mesa-Bains, A. (2006). *Homegrown: Engaged cultural criticism.* South End Press.

Houshmand, S., Spanierman, L. B., & De Stephano, J. (2017). Racial microaggressions: A primer with implications for counseling practice. *International Journal of Advanced Counselling, 39*, 203–216.

Kaur, V. (2021). *See no stranger: A memoir and manifesto of revolutionary love.* One World.

Kim, C. J. (1999). The racial triangulation of Asian Americans. *Politics & Society, 27*(1), 105–138.

Landa, M. H. (2012) Deconstructing black history month: Three African American boys' exploration of identity. *Multicultural Perspectives, 14*(1), 11–17.

Lee, R. T., Perez, A. D., Boykin, C. M., & Mendoza-Denton, R. (2019). On the prevalence of racial discrimination in the United States. *PLoS ONE, 14*(1), 1–16.

MacDonald, D. B., & Hudson, G. (2012). The genocide question and Indian residential schools in Canada. *Canadian Journal of Political Science/Revue Canadienne de Science Politique, 45*(2), 427–449.

Massey, D. S. (2015). The legacy of the 1968 Fair Housing Act. *Sociological Forum, 30*(S1), 571–588.

Matsuda, G. (1990). "Only the beginning": Continuing the fight for empowerment. *Amerasia Journal, 16*(1), 159–169.

Maynard, R. (2017). *Policing black lives: State violence in Canada from slavery to the present.* Fernwood Publishing.

Munroe, T. (2021). How to curb anti-black racism in Canadian schools. *The Conversation.* Retrieved March 28, 2023, from https://theconversation.com/how-to-curb-anti-black-racism-in-canadian-schools-150489

Museus, S. D. (2013). *Asian American students in higher education.* Routledge.

Natapoff, A. (1995). Trouble in paradise: Equal protection and the dilemma of interminority group conflict. *Stanford Law Review, 47*(5), 1059–1096.

Noh, E. (2018). Terror as usual: The role of the model minority myth in Asian American women's suicidality. *Women & Therapy, 41*(3–4), 316–338.

Oates, S. B. (2013). *Let the trumpet sound: A life of Martin Luther King, Jr.* Harper Perennial.

O'Donnell, K., Ewart, J., & Chrzanowski, A. (2018). "Don't freak we're Sikh" – A study of the extent to which Australian journalists and the Australian public wrongly associate Sikhism with Islam. *Religions, 9*(10), 319, 1–16.

Pierce, C. M., Carew, J., Pierce-Gonzalez, D., & Willis, D. (1978). An experiment in racism: TV commercials. In C. Pierce (Ed.), *Television and education* (pp. 62–88). Sage Publications.

Pyke, K. D. (2010). What is internalized racial oppression and why don't we study it? Acknowledging racism's hidden injuries. *Sociological Perspectives, 53*, 551–572.

Restoule, K. (2013). *An overview of the Indian residential school system.* Written by the Union of Ontario Indians based on research compiled by Karen Restoule. Creative Impressions.

Roberts, T., & Andrews, D. C. (2013). A critical race analysis of the gaslighting against African American teachers' considerations for recruitment and retention. In D. C. Andrews (Ed.), *Contesting the myth of a "post racial" era: The continued significance of race in U.S. education (black Studies and Critical Thinking)* (1st ed, pp. 69–94). Peter Lang.

Shams, T. (2020). Successful yet precarious: South Asian Muslim Americans, Islamophobia, and the model minority myth. *Sociological Perspectives, 63*(4), 653–669.

Shiao, J., & Woody, A. (2021). The meaning of "racism". *Sociological Perspectives, 64*(4), 495–517.

Sidhu, D. S. (2013). Lessons on terrorism and mistaken identity from Oak Creek, with a coda on the Boston marathon bombings. *Columbia Law Review Sidebar*, *113*, 76–87.

Simeon, T. (2010). *Safe drinking water in First Nations communities*. Parliamentary Information and Research Services, Library of Parliament Publication No. 08-43-E.

Singh, A. A. (2019). *Racial healing handbook: Practical activities to help you challenge privilege, confront systemic racism, and engage in collective healing*. New Harbinger Publications.

Sodhi, P. K. (2017). *Exploring immigrant and sexual minority mental health: Reconsidering multiculturalism*. Routledge.

Sojonky, T. (2010). *A self-study: Being a white psychologist in an Indian world*. Peter Lang International Academic Publishers.

Statistics Canada. (2019). *Diversity of black population in Canada: An overview*. Retrieved March 30, 2023, from www150.statcan.gc.ca/n1/en/pub/89-657-x/89-657-x2019002-eng.pdf?st=j0qEq2yM

Statistics Canada. (2021). *A snapshot: Status First Nations people in Canada*. Retrieved October 22, 2021, from www150.statcan.gc.ca/n1/pub/41-20-0002/412000022021001-eng.html

Sue, D. W., Capodilupo, C. M., Torino, G. C., Bucceri, J. M., Holder, A. M., Nadal, K. L., & Esquilin, M. (2007). Racial microaggressions in everyday life: Implications for clinical practice. *American Psychologist*, *62*, 271–286.

Tobias, H., & Joseph, A. (2020). Sustaining systemic racism through psychological gaslighting: Denials of racial profiling and justifications of carding by police utilizing local news media. *Race and Justice*, *10*(4), 424–455.

Viruell-Fuentes, E. A., Miranda, P. Y., & Abdulrahim, S. (2012). More than culture: Structural racism, intersectionality theory, and immigrant health. *Social Science & Medicine*, *75*, 2099–2106.

Wilkerson, I. (2020). *Caste: The origins of our discontents*. Random House.

Winters, M. F. (2020). *Black fatigue: How racism erodes the mind, body, and spirit*. Berrett-Koehler Publishers, Inc.

Yi, V., Mac, J., Na, V. S., Venturanza, R. J., Museus, S. D., Buenavista, T. L., & Pendakur, S. L. (2020). Toward an anti-imperialistic critical race analysis of the model minority myth. *Review of Educational Research*, *90*(4), 542–579.

Yi, V., & Museus, S. D. (2015). Model minority myth. In A. D. Smith, X. Hou, J. Stone, R. Dennis & P. Rizova (Eds.), *The Wiley Blackwell encyclopedia of race, ethnicity, and nationalism* (pp. 1–2). John Wiley & Sons, Ltd.

Chapter 6

Mental Health Implications and Developing an Anti-Racist Stance

This chapter clarifies mental health implications of racism, anti-racist practices, consistent allyship (productive versus performative), and supporting solidarity. The chapter culminates with insight about the need for land acknowledgements.

Racism and Mental Health

In both the literature and my clinical work, BIPOC clients have expressed the long-term effects and challenges racism has had on their overall wellbeing and the precautions that they have adopted to live safely in the Western culture (Meyer & Zane, 2013; Spence et al., 2016; Williams, 2020).

Mental health concerns can present differently in clients depending on how they are either epitomized or hidden in the client's ancestral culture. By listening to the client's past narrative and gathering background history, this reflective process can bring light to mental health symptoms that were deemed non-existent during diverse parts of the client's life (Sodhi, 2017). With the normalization of mental health and the intent to make therapy inviting and accessible for BIPOC, we are seeing increased representation of BIPOC within our therapeutic spaces. As therapists, it is critical to understand the cultural needs of our clients. There is a call for inclusive and intersectional mental healthcare for BIPOC individuals. Being further aware of the client's intersectionality will inform and structure their treatment plan accordingly (Collins & Bilge, 2016).

Some of the more researched mental health diagnoses related to experiencing either racism or oppression are anxiety, depression, chronic stress, substance use disorders, suicidality, PTSD, and intergenerational trauma (Paradies et al., 2015). As researched in *The First Nations Regional Health Survey* (FNIGC, 2018), which was administered between 2015 and 2017 and studied wellness within the First Nations communities, racism also brought on phobias, obsessive-compulsive disorder, panic

DOI: 10.4324/9781003216568-9

disorders, bipolar disorder, and mania in Indigenous peoples. Visible and invisible barriers prevent BIPOC clients from seeking help for these mental health issues; the next section details how one might challenge these barriers.

Importance of Accessing Mental Health Services

Consistent with post-migration concerns, BIPOC may experience further stressors around the migration process and isolation in the host country, employment and financial issues, developing a bicultural identity, and loss of family networks which inadvertently may affect their self-confidence and increase mental health symptoms (Sodhi, 2017). There are relevant barriers to obtaining help from mental health practitioners:

- Financial limitations regarding service fees/costs.
- Unfamiliarity with mental health issues and the North American healthcare system.
- Cultural and social stigma associated with speaking about issues outside of the family.
- Structural racism, racial microaggressions, and model minority myth stereotypes.
- Lack of representation and scarcity of culturally responsive mental health practitioners.
- Confidentiality concerns and fear of other community members learning about accessing therapy.
- Communication/language issues and the inability to express oneself clearly in host culture language.
- Experiencing historical or political repression, leaving BIPOC feeling helpless and speechless in talk therapy.

Cultural shame and avoiding symptoms could impede accessing mental health services. Maintaining family image, not bringing dishonour to the family, preferring to seek help in another community, and fear of being seen attending therapy are also relevant obstacles (Das & Kemp, 1997; Sodhi, 2019).

Making Therapy Accessible to BIPOC

A former student of mine wisely expressed that "therapy is political and considered a Western luxury or capitalist commodity." That is, therapy is typically eurocentric and mostly affordable to those who have financial resources or workplace benefits. As practitioners, part of our role is to assist clients in overcoming challenges to accessing culturally responsive services. Earlier in my career as a psychotherapist, one of my clinical supervisors shared an invaluable quote about the messaging behind seeking therapy; that is, "the whole point of going to therapy is to get out of therapy." Over the years, I have expressed this sentiment to clients; as a result, they have felt informed, confident, and therefore immersed themselves in the therapeutic process. Clients essentially "do the work," develop better symptom management, and overcome barriers. There are, however, select clients who encounter a multitude of barriers upon commencing therapy. What if starting therapy is their biggest barrier?

How can we advocate for sustainable therapeutic accessibility for BIPOC communities? By offering free consultations; extending sliding scales; normalizing and destigmatizing therapy; working from an anti-oppressive lens; discussing the therapeutic process with special attention given to limits to confidentiality; providing psychoeducation about mental health; and involving the community in care, clients may feel empowered, seen, heard, and respected rather than stigmatized in a therapeutic context.

Locating an Anti-Racist and Culturally Responsive Therapist

One of the most discouraging barriers to accessing therapy is finding a compatible therapist. According to the American Psychological Association (2021), most psychologists are white (86%) and only a small percentage are racialized (14%). This disparity may impede clients' initiatives to find a therapist who is the right fit for them; such a therapist may be someone who integrates Eastern ideologies and healing practices into their work. It is integral for practitioners to be knowledgeable about BIPOC communities, cultural backgrounds, therapeutic presenting problems, traditions, values, and beliefs, as well as the importance of community care and self-care.

This list unveils some of the more prevalent topics that are discussed by my BIPOC clients; when the topic is about a specific presenting problem or situational stressor, often that stressor is steeped in a pool of racism and trauma that is much harder for the client to articulate.

- Acculturation stress
- Migratory mental health concerns
- Post-traumatic stress disorder (PTSD)
- Intergenerational trauma
- Racial trauma

- Internalized racism
- Cultural shaming and guilt
- Anger, rage, or aggression
- Cultural and racial discrimination
- Cross-cultural grief
- Imposter syndrome
- Cultural burnout
- Extended family matters
- Intergenerational conflict
- Cultural existential crises
- Codependency and attachment issues
- Assertiveness and resiliency training
- Negotiating cultural boundaries
- Workplace discrimination and adjustment

Prior to starting the therapeutic or counselling process in a private practice setting, a variety of questions could be asked by the therapist and client during a complimentary 15–30 minute consultation. This dialogue helps determine therapeutic compatibility and alignment of visions concerning treatment planning. If a free consultation is not available, clients might be able to locate responses on prospective therapists' websites. I am often asked these questions during a consultation:

1. What is your cultural/racial background and how does it inform your work?
2. What are your anti-oppressive and trauma-informed approaches? Which culturally responsive theoretical orientations do you lean into?
3. What is your training and reason for pursuing this career trajectory?
4. What is your knowledge and experience working with a _____ (specific cultural/racial group)?
5. What is your awareness and experience working with BIPOC who have encountered racism?
6. What is your comfort level regarding talking about topics such as colonialism, systemic oppression, and white privilege?
7. What approaches do you use to address issues such as racism and discrimination?
8. How have you dismantled various forms of societal oppressive systems?

There is evidently a demand for therapists who are culturally responsive and adhere to anti-oppressive practices.

Community Care

Community care is a decolonized approach to healing which is more racially equitable and accessible. Community care could be considered more than default individualistic Western approaches. Care is woven into the communities in which BIPOC have been socialized and have social networks. Community care involves creating community connections and intentional actions so that everyone can benefit from collective healing (Cummins, 2020). Within the Sikh faith, the Punjabi term *seva* lends itself well with regards to community care. Seva is the Sanskrit word "to serve." It is also a form of selfless act and promotes intersectional equality (Kaur, 2021; Sodhi, 2022).

Community care is self-care; it requires time to rest and heal so that members can take care of one another. It is based on collectivist ideologies whereby communities help communities via circle of care, sharing/healing circles, community healing/solidarity vigils, community health workers, daily or weekly phone, text, or virtual check-ins, preparing meals for community members in need, volunteering for a cause, or becoming a productive ally. We clearly noticed the prominence of community care during the COVID-19 pandemic, as individuals were unable to connect with their families domestically or abroad due to the restrictions that were placed as a global whole.

Overcoming Racial Oppression, Healing, and Becoming Resilient

Harro's framework, *The Cycle of Socialization,* illustrates that how we are socialized influences our perceptions about oppressive systems and power (Harro, 2000). The evolution of decentring systemic racism can be examined using main concepts from Figure 6.1:

1. At the *Core*, there may be initial resistance, reluctance, and ambivalence about race-related concepts; norms, values, beliefs, stereotypes, generalizations, and biases are potentially formulated through white and colonial lenses.
2. *The Begining* represents a clean slate, where individuals experience no consciousness, blame, or guilt. They are unaware of their cultural beliefs/values/traditions as well as their biases, stereotypes, and prejudices thus far.
3. *First Socialization* involves the individuals, typically family, peers, or mentors who introduce and reinforce diverse constructs.
4. *Institutional and Cultural Socialization* involve media, schools, and other systems. These beliefs become normalized, ingrained, and accepted by society.

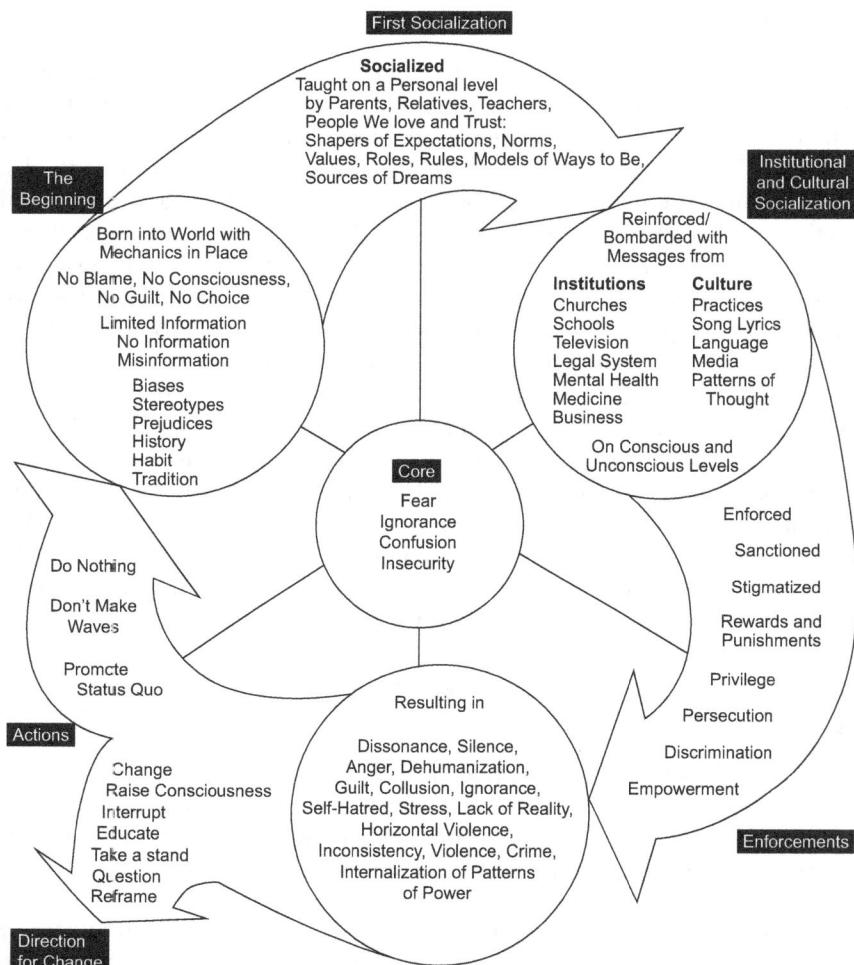

Figure 6.1 The cycle of socialization (Harro, 2000) – with permission from Taylor and Francis Group

5. Additional *Enforcements* implicates ways of conforming and non-conforming. Stigma, rewards, and punishments further solidify what has been established by earlier socialization experiences.
6. *Results* take the form of internal feelings and social standing that are twofold: Abnormal (i.e., shame, silence, and isolation) and Normal (i.e., confidence, security, autonomy).

7. *Direction for Change* refers to opportunities to break *The Cycle of Socialization*. To create spaces safe for BIPOC, some directions for change are:

- Dismantling positions of power, privilege, and oppression.
- Overcoming coloniality, which is the "long-standing patterns of power that emerged as a result of colonialism, but that define culture, labor, intersubjective relations, and knowledge production well beyond the strict limits of colonial administrations" (Bhatia & Priya, 2021, p. 423).
- Recognizing the significance of staying current in our language and messaging while working with BIPOC clients.
- Silencing colonial and eurocentric therapeutic approaches and replacing them with more inclusive practices.
- Identifying and decolonizing academia by way of BIPOC representation and implementing culturally responsive curricula.
- Amplifying and building awareness, allyship, and solidarity for BIPOC communities.

8. *Actions* are behaviours that can either perpetuate or break *The Cycle of Socialization*. Actions that correspond to the aforementioned *Direction for Change* include the eradication of the colonial white supremist intergenerational cycle by reinforcing and developing an anti-racist stance.

The next section demonstrates the efforts and information required to shift from being a performative ally to a productive ally.

Developing an Anti-Racist Stance: What Is Required?

"You have to act as if it were possible to radically transform the world. And you have to do it all the time," proclaimed Angela Davis during a lecture at *Southern Illinois University* (Davis, 2014). There is no precise road map to anti-racist practices. With this movement in full force, part of what needs to transpire is the unlearning of certain thoughts, feelings, and behaviours that contribute to our distorted perceptions of humanity. We need to constantly check and re-evaluate our choice points and biases. Choice points provide opportunities to make socially constructive decisions that can influence racial equity and unbiased outcomes. I have learned that racism did not only evolve from nationalism; racism could be a result of our negative self-perception that is projected onto others. We must tap into some inner work rather than accessing Western conventional psychology, which is more colonial and individualistic. With Eastern approaches, one is encouraged to look within and source answers that surround us. Until there is resolve regarding these concerns, racism, hate, and rage will continue to occupy our minds, communities, societies, and global world.

One of the objectives of this chapter is to provide a framework that abolishes racism and prejudice towards BIPOC communities. Drawing from a health equity perspective, we must keep in mind the necessity of enforcement, new legislation, and advocacy; we should also reduce residual damage, spread awareness, and change white attitudes to successfully eliminate racism (Braveman et al., 2022). But do these Western ideologies exude undertones of eurocentric beliefs and power dynamics? Is history repeating itself? Irrespective, the racism that exists warrants undermining through further discourse about the root cause of colonial racism and systemic elements that influence these Western thought processes (i.e., enforcement, legislation, advocacy, and affirmative action). From here, I turn to Mahatma Gandhi's principle, *Satyagraha*, translated as "holding on to truth" or "insistence on truth" (Sodhi, 1988, p. 1). This principle consists of three beliefs: *satya* (truth), *ahimsa* (openness, honesty, and non-injury), and *tapasya* (patience and altruism) (Sodhi, 1988). These concepts can support and empower anti-racist work and improve mental health services for BIPOC individuals. This can be accomplished by mobilizing communities and following up on social justice causes that inspire healing. Below are other initiatives to overcome racism within particular ecosystems:

- Home: facilitate purposeful and intergenerational conversations about racism, timely and relevant definitions, awareness of media representation, and explore what is being individually internalized by each family member.
- Academic setting: enhance classrooms with culturally relevant policies, curricula, and teaching practices.
- Community: augment social justice, care, cohesiveness, and inclusivity as qualities within neighbours.
- Host culture: endorse positive interactions between BIPOC and cultural/ethnic/racial communities and involvement in annual cultural celebrations.

The word *ally* is occasionally misused or misrepresented in several contexts. To further understand the steps associated with becoming an *ally*, performative and productive allyship must be differentiated from one another. Central to allyship is putting words (or intentions) into actions. A conflict may occur when cultural values and beliefs are inaccurately conveyed such that they cause more harm than good within society. We see such misunderstandings with cultural appropriation, erasure, and the dissemination of racial stereotypes that somehow appear in our therapeutic environments. These stereotypes can show up as a presenting issue or in therapists who have not explored their personal biases. Anchored in the above-mentioned content pertaining to anti-racist strategies, Figure 6.2

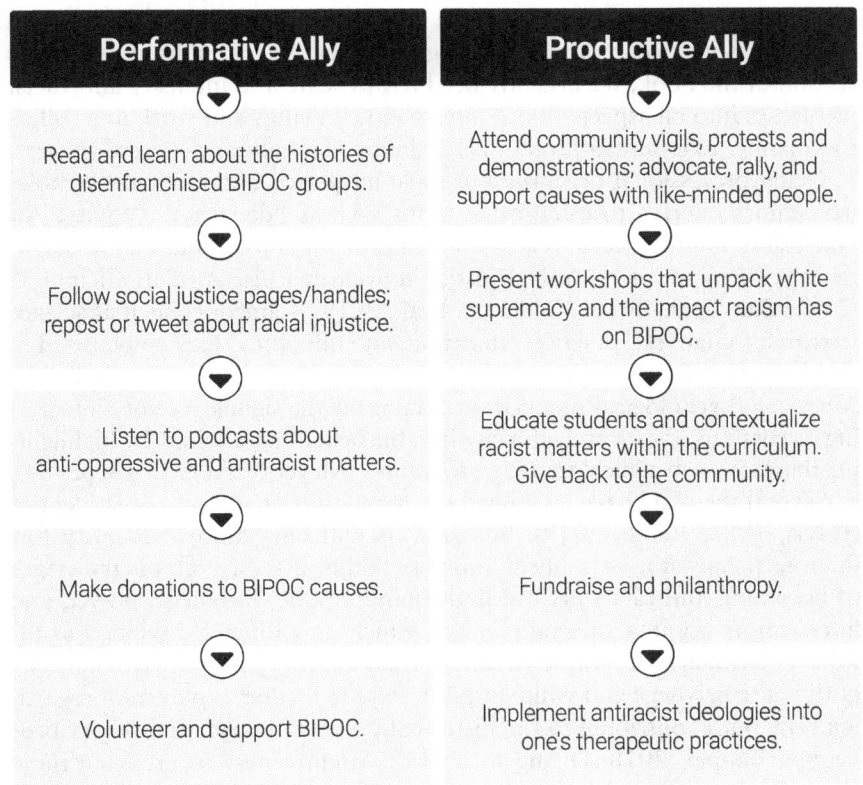

Figure 6.2 Performative versus productive ally hallmarks

illuminates how a racially informed individual can shift from being a performative ally to a productive ally.

There are varied pathways towards becoming a productive ally; it is important to cultivate a community that appreciates the progression towards capacity building upon this intention (Akbar, 2020). Analogous to music, as we move from a decrescendo to a crescendo, or from a silenced voice to an amplified voice, we could attract more interest in joining a movement to foster and support accountability and follow-through in one's actions.

The subsequent section outlines options for sustaining anti-racist practices, identifying next steps, and recourse.

Sustaining Anti-Racist Practices

As defined by Singh (2019), "Antiracist refers to people who are actively seeking not only to raise their consciousness about race and racism, but also to take action when they see racial power inequities in everyday life"

(p. 87). As an anti-racist, one should strive to be congruent and consistent in their actions to end racism. Highlighting what has been discussed in this section of the book, we urgently need to advocate and intensify anti-racist ideologies into all aspects of our intersectional beings and work in a collective manner to ensure anti-racism is maintained in differing societal spheres.

Many professional organizations have integrated anti-racist deliverables (sometimes referred to using other terms such as "diversity," "equity," or "inclusion") in their calls to action to support BIPOC communities in alignment with many of the social justice movements discussed in Chapter 5 (Abdel-Baki et al., 2020; Hollinrake et al., 2019). Categories such as science (research initiatives), practice, education, and advocacy were emphasized in the Canadian Psychological Association's (2020) initiatives. Similarly, the American Psychological Association documents the significance of "integrating discussions of race and ethnicity into the field of psychology by highlighting these issues in clinical training programs" (Meyer & Zane, 2013, p. 884).

Several theorists have examined the formation of an anti-racist identity (Davis, 1983; Kendi, 2019); however, as with any kind of identity formation, it may not be a linear process (Sodhi, 2017). Preliminary stages of becoming anti-racist involve understanding one's privilege, power, and intersectionality in a societal context, which may differ for white and BIPOC individuals (Bryant & Arrington, 2022; Singh, 2020). For example, both white privilege and white fragility require further exploration regarding how both contribute to the historical cycles of racism and power brokerage (Bhopal, 2018; DiAngelo, 2018). Attentiveness to breaking these cycles by becoming an educator, advocate, or racial ally helps cease all forms of racism. Racial stamina encourages white individuals to reflect upon their racial biases and consciousness by having intentional conversation and learning from BIPOC (Grzanka et al., 2020). By building racial stamina, white individuals move from coping with racism to mitigating it via anti-racist practices. Evolving as such will generate moments of confusion, regret, healing, and acceptance for white individuals that can be resolved by respecting diverse cultural spaces.

While I was teaching graduate level courses about cultural diversity, enrolled students were asked to complete the Implicit Association Test (IAT) produced by Harvard University (Project Implicit, 2011). These students learned more about their preferences, associations, subconscious biases, and stereotypes towards diverse populations (Beckles-Raymond, 2020). Referencing these test scores, I have had invigorating conversation with my students concerning the necessity of applying theory (performative) into practice (productive) regarding anti-racist identity development, which manifests itself by means of experiential learning. Such learning can invite reading anti-racist literature, attending cultural events or festivals, travelling, visiting cultural enclaves in larger urban centres, reaching out to BIPOC friends and family in times of need and providing support, and learning from friends, colleagues, or classmates by joining in their lived experience and/or familial cultural traditions (Harper, 2022). Through these lived experience, one learns about the attributes of various communities. It is imperative to immerse, learn, and celebrate diverse cultures and their messages so that we can genuinely be present for BIPOC.

On the other end of the BIPOC/white binary, for BIPOC, precluding interminority racism is fundamental in developing an anti-racist identity and acknowledging the severity that white supremacy and internalized racism continues to have on BIPOC (Pyke, 2010). To cultivate an anti-racist identity, BIPOC need to overcome ethnocentrism (the belief that one's ethnicity is superior to another) and "unlearn internalized whiteness" (Singh, 2020, p. 1116). It suggests BIPOC working together to decentre the historical white supremist colonial beliefs that plague BIPOC's sense of unity (Cortland et al., 2017). BIPOC communities can rally as a collective, defy racial violence, and actualize healing that does not subscribe to proximity privilege (to members of the host country) (Saad, 2020); rather, this healing resembles standing together in solidarity, showing up for each other, and overcoming mutual fears.

Based on anti-racist constructs and content from Chapters 5 and 6, the reverse pyramid shown in Figure 6.3 captures potential steps towards becoming anti-racist ally.

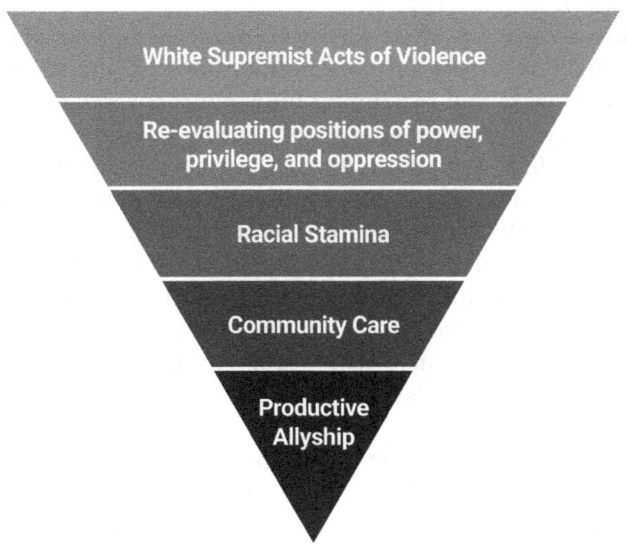

Figure 6.3 Anti-racist inverted pyramid

During the process of developing an anti-racist identity, we migrate from a scarcity mindset of denying and enabling white supremist acts of violence to achieving a growth or abundance mindset by observing positions of power, privilege, and oppression, engaging in racial stamina, understanding the significance of community care, and becoming a productive ally. As a collective society focussing on a mutual cause, the production of current research to improve the betterment of BIPOC is imperative. One cannot stay silent about systemic and institutional issues, racism, and racial trauma. One should show up, however possible, and learn to be accountable for their actions. Allyship cannot be context or population specific, nor can it entail choosing when to partipate or dedicate to a cause.

Allyship is not about coping with or managing the repercussions of a system; it is about eradicating it and acknowledging the colonial injustice that invaded one's psyche. From here, one can step back further and take stock of the eurocentric, imperialist conditioning such as national holidays.

Cancel Culture

The term "cancel culture" has existed within our vernacular for years and has received recent popularity on social media. By definition, "cancel culture is a phenomenon where individuals transgressing norms are called out and ostracised on social media and other venues by members of the public" (Saint-Louis, 2021, p. 1).

Over the last decade, there has been immense uproar about cancel culture and/or boycotting national holidays (e.g., Canada Day, July 4, and Columbus Day) and reclaiming Indigenous sovereignty. Many Canadians were apprehensive about celebrating Canada Day on July 1, 2021, after the discovery of numerous unmarked Indigenous children's graves and genocide. How can multicultural/immigrant/BIPOC feel safe in a country that supported residential schools? Canada Day can be conflicting, particularly for immigrants leaving a colonized land to migrate to another colonized land. Therefore, I felt as if my patriotic connection to Canada was being compromised, which led me to naming the problem with the historical meaning of Canada Day. I wrote the following reflections that day:

> *It is not a year to celebrate. I feel betrayed, unsafe, and misinformed about this country my parents immigrated to 60 years ago. Yesterday, I felt vulnerable when I saw a pick-up truck with two large Canadian flags, spotted on my drive home. Later in the day, on my walk with*

my partner, we talked about how there is still a need to assimilate and conform to the colonial ways; whether it is through internalized racism and abandoning one's culture and language or changing one's appearance and looking more Western. My parents dealt with these hardships as they immigrated to a town in Northern Alberta where turbaned men and sari clad women were unheard of. My father's narrative included a very heart-wrenching experience of removing his turban, shaving his beard, and cutting his hair so that he could obtain employment and "fit" into the North American culture. In actuality, he did not feel a sense of belonging in either culture and was treated differently by his family for abandoning his turban upon returning back to India for an annual visit. To this day he is regretful for altering his appearance to seek approval from the host culture.

The revelation of children's bodies further enhanced my recognition that I am living on colonized land that was previously inhabited and stolen from the Indigenous peoples (Fonseca, 2020). Colonization is ubiquitous and traumatizes those whose rights are taken away from them. With these sentiments in mind, let us proceed into a decolonized and re-Indigenized discussion on the messaging about land acknowledgements.

Land Acknowledgements

The "94 Calls to Action" in the *Truth and Reconciliation Report* underscore the need to appreciate and address the stolen lands and territories that are being inhabited (Commission of Canada, 2015). Thusly, we are elevating and honouring the Indigenous ancestors, voices, heritage, history, and identity. A land acknowledgement or Indigenous affirmation is a succinct declaration customarily shared at the beginning of an event identifying the Indigenous territory where the events are being held. The content of the land acknowledgement offers information about the names of the First Nations and the specific area and treaties that govern the region. It concludes with expressing gratitude for the land and recognizing the hardships and injustice experiences by the First Nations, Métis, and Inuit peoples (Canadian context) (Stewart-Ambo & Yang, 2021). For example:

I am grateful and honoured to be working on the ancestral lands of the First Nation, Métis, and Inuit peoples. I recognize that this book was written on the unceded territory of the Algonquin Anishinaabe Nation. I also acknowledge that the applicable treaties for this region are referred to as the Peace and Friendship Treaties. I reaffirm my responsibility to increase awareness and understanding of First Nations, Métis, and Inuit peoples and colonial legacy, and commit to strengthening my relationship with Indigenous peoples throughout Canada.

More information about land acknowledgements in North America can be found at: https://native-land.ca/ and https://nativegov.org/news/a-guide-to-indigenous-land-acknowledgment/.

Traditionally, land acknowledgements are an Indigenous protocol that identify areas and regions they would visit and recognize the relationship and historical context between the people and inhabited land. Due to colonialism, land acknowledgements are communicated in present tense as a reminder of the hurt and trauma that occurred within these communities. It is our role to "give back," respect, carry forward this tradition, and educate others about the repercussions of these colonial actions (Robinson et al., 2019; Tuck & Yang, 2012).

Lastly, to complete this chapter, here are some strategies to honour Indigenous communities and build and sustain meaningful relationships with their people (Statistics Canada, 2021; Stewart-Ambo & Yang, 2021):

- Reflect upon how the ideology of "Land Back" resonates with you.
- Familiarize yourself with the respected territory treaties and titles.
- Establish trust and demonstrate transparency and respect toward Indigenous causes.
- Appreciate literature and watch movies produced by and starring Indigenous actors.
- Recognize and know the history of the "stolen" land we inhabit.
- Explore the meaning of Orange Shirt Day by reading Phyllis Webstad's narrative.
- Understand and listen to the history, hardships, barriers, and intergenerational trauma endured by residential school survivors and those who did not return home.
- Commemorate and integrate First Nations, Métis, and Inuit voices and teachings in academic settings; include Indigenous content and Indigeneity into the curriculum.
- Honour residential school survivors through sacred ceremonies and memorials.
- Enrol in a free Indigenous Canada course offered by the University of Alberta at: https://bit.ly/304HJKU
- Read the Truth and Reconciliation Report which offers "94 Calls to Action"; learn how to become a productive ally.

In the proceeding parts of this book, I discuss additional strategies to decolonize our therapeutic practices as well as how to integrate anti-racist practices into one's approach to therapy.

References

Abdel-Baki, R., Collaton, J., Courtice, E. L., Gayfer, B., Lee, S., Narvaez Linares, N. F., & Tang, K. T. Y. (2020). *Toward anti-racism in Canadian psychology: A call to action from the future of the field.* PsyArXiv.

Akbar, M. (2020). *Beyond ally: The pursuit to racial justice.* Publish Your Purpose Press.

American Psychological Association. (2021). *The psychology of hate crimes.* Retrieved August 25, 2021, from www.apa.org/advocacy/interpersonal-violence/hate-crimes

Beckles-Raymond, G. R. (2020). Implicit bias, (global) white ignorance, and bad faith: The problem of whiteness and anti-black racism. *Journal of Applied Philosophy, 37*(2), 169–189.

Bhatia, S., & Priya, K. R. (2021). Coloniality and psychology: From silencing to re-centering marginalized voices in postcolonial times. *Review of General Psychology, 25*(4), 422–436.

Bhopal, K. (2018). *White privilege: The myth of a post-racial society.* Policy Press.

Braveman, P. A., Arkin, E., Proctor, D., Kauh, T., & Holm, N. (2022). Systemic and structural racism: Definitions, examples, health damages, and approaches to dismantling. *Health Affairs, 41*(2), 171–178.

Bryant, T., & Arrington, E. D. (2022). *The antiracism handbook: Practical tools to shift your mindset and uproot racism in your life and community.* New Harbinger Publications Inc.

Canadian Psychological Association. (2020). *Open letter to the Canadian Psychological Association.* Canadian Psychological Association.

Collins, P. H., & Bilge, S. (2016). *Intersectionality: Key concepts.* Polity Press.

Commission of Canada. (2015). *Honouring the truth, reconciling the future, summary of the truth and reconciliation.* Commission of Canada.

Cortland, C. I., Craig, M. A., Shapiro, J. R., Richeson, J. A., Neel, R., & Goldstein, N. J. (2017). Solidarity through shared disadvantage: Highlighting shared experiences of discrimination improves relations between stigmatized groups. *Journal of Personality and Social Psychology, 113*(4), 547–567.

Cummins, I. (2020). *Mental health services and community care: A critical history.* Policy Press.

Das, A. K., & Kemp, S. (1997). Between two worlds: Counselling South Asian Americans. *Journal of Multicultural Counselling and Development, 25,* 23–33.

Davis, A. Y. (1983). *Women, race & class.* Vintage Books.

Davis, A. Y. (2014, February 13). Lecture delivered at Southern Illinois University, Carbondale.

DiAngelo, R. (2018). *White fragility: Why it's so hard for white people to talk about racism.* Beacon Press.

First Nations Information Governance Centre (FNIGC). (2018). *The first nations regional health survey phase 3, 1.* First Nations Information Governance Centre (FNIGC).

Fonseca, S. (2020). Institutional racism in Canada: Indigenous lived realities. *The Society: Sociology and Criminology Undergraduate Review, 5*(1), 50–59.

Grzanka, P. R., Frantell, K. A., & Fassinger, R. E. (2020). The white racial affect scale (WRAS): A measure of white guilt, shame, and negation. *The Counseling Psychologist, 48*(1), 47–77.

Harper, M. (2022). *10 steps to non-optical allyship*. Johns Hopkins Medicine, Office of Diversity, Inclusion and Health Equity.

Harro, B. (2000). The cycle of socialization. In M. Adams, W. Blumenfeld, R. Castaneda, H. Hackman, M. Peters & X. Zuniga (Eds.), *Readings for diversity and social justice* (pp. 15–20). Routledge.

Hollinrake, S., Hunt, G., Dix, H., & Wagner, A. (2019). Do we practice (or teach) what we preach? Developing a more inclusive learning environment to better prepare social work students for practice through improving the exploration of their different ethnicities within teaching, learning and assessment opportunities. *Social Work Education, 38*(5), 582–603.

Kaur, V. (2021). *See no stranger: A memoir and manifesto of revolutionary love*. One World.

Kendi, I. X. (2019). *How to be an antiracist*. One World.

Meyer, O. L., & Zane, N. (2013). The influence of race and ethnicity in the client's experiences of mental health treatment. *Journal of Community Psychology, 41*(7), 884–901.

Paradies, Y., Ben, J., Denson, N., Elias, A., Priest, N., Pieterse, A., Gupta, A., Kelaher, M., & Gee, G. (2015). Racism as a determinant of health: A systematic review and meta-analysis. *PLoS ONE, 10*(9), e0138511.

Project Implicit. (2011). Retrieved March 23, 2023, from https://implicit.harvard.edu/implicit/Study?tid=-1

Pyke, K. D. (2010). What is internalized racial oppression and why don't we study it? Acknowledging racism's hidden injuries. *Sociological Perspectives, 53*, 551–572.

Robinson, D., Hill, K. J. C., Ruffo, A. G., Couture, S., & Ravensbergen, L. C. (2019). Rethinking the practice and performance of Indigenous land acknowledgement. *Canadian Theatre Review, 177*(1), 20–30.

Saad, L. F. (2020). *Me and white supremacy: Combat racism, change the world, and become a good ancestor*. Sourcebooks, Inc.

Saint-Louis, H. (2021). Understanding cancel culture: Normative and unequal sanctioning. *First Monday, 26*(7), 1–17.

Singh, A. A. (2019). *Racial healing handbook: Practical activities to help you challenge privilege, confront systemic racism, and engage in collective healing*. New Harbinger Publications.

Singh, A. A. (2020). Building a counseling psychology of liberation: The path behind us, under us, and before us. *The Counseling Psychologist, 48*(8), 1109–1130.

Sodhi, P. K. (2017). *Exploring immigrant and sexual minority mental health: Reconsidering multiculturalism*. Routledge.

Sodhi, P. K. (2019). Diversity and identity formation therapy: An integrative model for immigrants and sexual minorities. Discussion forum presented at the *Canadian Psychological Association conference*. Halifax, Nova Scotia, May 31–June 2, 2019.

Sodhi, P. (2022). Trauma-informed care for BIPOC communities. Speaker series hosted by the *Canadian Counselling and Psychotherapy Association*, November 16, 2022.

Sodhi, S. K. (1988). *Mahatma Gandhi: A psycho dynamic critique*. Commonwealth Publishers.

Spence, N. D., Wells, S., Graham, K., & George, J. (2016). Racial discrimination, cultural resilience, and stress. *The Canadian Journal of Psychiatry, 61*(5), 298–307.

Statistics Canada. (2021). *A snapshot: Status First Nations people in Canada.* Retrieved October 22, 2021, from www150.statcan.gc.ca/n1/pub/41-20-0002/412000022021001-eng.html

Stewart-Ambo, T., & Yang, K. W. (2021). Beyond land acknowledgment in settler institutions. *Social Text, 39*(1(146)), 21–46.

Tuck, E., & Yang, W. K. (2012). Decolonization is not a metaphor. *Decolonization: Indigeneity, Education & Society, 1*(1), 1–40.

Williams, M. T. (2020). Microaggressions: Clarification, evidence, and impact. *Perspectives on Psychological Science, 15*(1), 3–26.

Part 3

Listening to Intergenerational BIPOC Narratives

Introduction

The following five composite BIPOC narratives are based on real life accounts from clients, students, colleagues, peers, and people in the media who have shared their vulnerabilities in diverse spaces over the years; yet, the details and stories have been woven to protect the anonymity of these resilient individuals. As mentioned in the introduction, these narratives set the tone for an extensive analysis in the form of case conceptualizations and treatment plans in Part 4 of this book. These stories represent the Black, Indigenous, South Asian, Latine, and Asian communities.

Jamal

Jamal is a 21-year-old black heterosexual cisgender male. His father's family are involuntary immigrants from Nigeria and fled the country in 1969 during the *Nigerian Civil War.* Jamal's mother's ancestry dates to the years of enslavement and being a part of the *American Civil Rights* Movement in the 1960s. Both sides of the family experienced an abundance of intergenerational and racial trauma.

His family currently resides in Detroit, where his father works in a car factory and his mother teaches music to neighbourhood children. Jamal's father has dealt with plenty of racial discrimination in the workplace and was told that he is "worthless and lazy." Jamal is the eldest of four children; his youngest brother has been accused of other forms of crimes and was wrongfully incarcerated. Throughout Jamal's childhood, he was bullied by his white peers. He heard stories of his relatives being mistreated and abused by members of the host culture, while simultaneously feeling othered and experiencing racism, criminalization, discrimination, and barriers towards employment opportunities.

Given this unsettling past, Jamal made efforts to break barriers and cycles of trauma for subsequent familial generations. During his schooling,

DOI: 10.4324/9781003216568-10

he became interested in learning more about black leaders such as Dr. Martin Luther King, Jr., Malcom X, and Barack Obama and aspired to be a lawyer or political leader one day. He participated in several *Black Lives Matter* events. He learned how to play the piano and became a varsity soccer player. He was a straight A student and received several scholarships to attend prestigious universities. With reservation and fear of being a target of hate crimes, he eventually accepted an offer from a predominantly white Ivy League university. He decided to pursue a political science major, with plans to attend law school where he hopes to represent discrimination and harassment cases. Jamal had a clear academic and professional future ahead of him.

One evening after class, while walking through an obscure part of campus, he was stopped by two white police officers. They questioned why he was on this exclusive campus. He stated that he was a senior student and was simply walking back to his dormitory to study for his upcoming midterms. They did not believe him and asked him for proof of student ID. As one police officer examined his ID with a flashlight, the other moved behind him and grabbed his arms and restrained him. He discreetly whispered in Jamal's ear, "Niggers don't belong here!"

Jamal was shocked but knew not to fight the police officer. He had heard about his uncles/ancestors who were shunned out of restaurants and busses in the 1950s and 1960s, chose to fight back, and were further harmed by police officers. The tormenting continued with mocking, derogatory/racist name calling, and then each police officer started to take turns punching Jamal first in the arm and then in the stomach, until he fell to the ground. The police officer holding Jamal's student ID threw it next to Jamal and told him to tell his *people* to stop robbing banks.

Jamal was in shock and disbelief to have become a victim of police brutality, particularly in his aspiration of being a cycle breaker. This horrific hate crime will forever be etched in his racialized psyche; correspondingly, it will also serve as a catalyst to spread awareness and rally like-minded individuals to dismantle white supremist acts of violence. Jamal reported this event, yet he was not taken seriously and further experienced racial gaslighting and microaggressions from the manager of campus security. It was only when he spoke with a racialized dean that his voice was heard, and consistent changes were made. This validation initially helped with Jamal's healing process; however, years of intergenerational trauma that were strategically and genetically stored in his nervous system were activated (Winters, 2020). He was in dire need of receiving culturally affirming therapeutic support to process past trauma and the police brutality event.

Mikom

Mikom (formerly known as Mike) is a 32-year-old two-spirit Mi'kmaq individual whose pronouns are they/them. They are a member of the *K'jipuktuk* (Halifax, Nova Scotia) 2SLGBTQQIA+ community. Mi'kmaq is the word for *people* and is the most prominent Indigenous community in the Maritime provinces of Canada (Tesar, 2022). Over the years, several generations of Mi'kmaq continue to encounter forced assimilation, cultural genocide, and colonial and intergenerational trauma.

Their story of systemic oppression started around seventeenth century when their people first experienced colonization. It was the Europeans (French and English) who landed on the coast of Nova Scotia, Canada, and claimed Mikom's family's territory. The Mi'kmaq chose to support the French and converted to Roman Catholicism. Yet there was some miscommunication, and in the end the British gained access to the land from the French. Due to the juxtaposition of perseverance and several peace agreements (between 1725 and 1761), Mikom's relatives were able to permanently reclaim their land.

From 1801 to 1821, Indian reserves were established throughout Nova Scotia. With the proclamation of the *Confederation* (1867) and the *Indian Civilization Act* (1876), the federal government created residential schools (see Chapter 5), attended by Mikom's ancestors. Multiple generations of Indigenous people were sent to the *Shubenacadie Indian Residential School* (between 1930 and 1967) where they were stripped away of their Indigenous identity. False promises were made to families indicating the return of their children; however, these children never returned to their parents. Instead, they suffered through internalized racism, abuse, and unfathomable trauma.

Mikom's grandmother attended the *Shubenacadie Indian Residential School* and shared her hardships of being told to assimilate to the Western ways. She was fortunate to have successfully escaped the residential school system and was in essence a cycle breaker who refused to send her children. This resistance, however, did not mask the mental health issues resulting from her time spent at the residential school. Mikom was socialized by their extended family who collectively lived on the *Glooscap* First Nations reserve, 68 kilometres away from Halifax. Mikom has two older sisters who left the reserve at the age of 18 and now live in Truro, Nova Scotia. From a young age, Mikom felt the repercussion of their grandmother's trauma as they witnessed her having severe panic attacks and episodes of mild psychosis. Mikom's parents are divorced, and Mikom has not seen their father since they were seven-years-old. Additionally, their mother was depressed throughout her lifetime.

Growing up on the reserve, Mikom was able to embody and appreciate Mi'kmaq culture. They participated in a variety of events and they believed strongly in the values and beliefs that were being instilled in them. They enjoyed painting as well as other creative endeavours and healing practices offered by community members. Around the age of 14, Mikom started questioning their sexuality and gender. They weren't sure about their identities. In fact, they were approached by another questioning teen on the reserve to go on a date together; Mikom declined due to the fear of the unknown. As the year continued, Mikom was able to talk with this person about their hesitations about dating and not being able to name their sexual orientation. Their friend introduced them to the concept of two-spirit: an Indigenous way of being that holds no barriers between cultural, general, sexual, and spiritual identity (Blue et al., 2015). A two-spirit person is said to encompass both a feminine and masculine spirit and is part of the 2SLGBTQQIA+ acronym. This term immediately resonated with Mikom, who follows the traditions and beliefs of a two-spirit individual while simultaneously trying to grapple with their past.

To cope, Mikom started drinking and smoking cannabis shortly after the age of 13 years. They were not sure how to deal with their extended family's centuries of intergenerational trauma and the impact it continues to have on their generation. In the past, they had tried speaking to the Elders on their reserve in hopes that there would be a chance to grieve these past familial events, process, heal, and move forward in a brave manner. While speaking to the Elder, they felt some relief for seeking help and understanding Indigenous healing practices, yet there was nominal assistance for overcoming their substance use, grieving their estranged father, and guilt for moving to Halifax, Nova Scotia, to be with other 2SLGBTQQIA+ community members. Mikom would like to comprehend their substance use disorder and learn about the abandonment wound that is creating personal obstacles in their life.

Prem

Prem is a 90-year-old South Asian heterosexual cisgender male who was born in Punjab, India. He is the youngest of six sons born between 1920 and 1933. His father was a hard-working teacher but also quite aloof; he used to physically punish Prem and his brothers to keep them in line. Prem was physically abused regardless of the reason, and some of his brothers were beaten to the point of unconsciousness. Even though Prem originated from a family of educators, his grandfather made moonshine; Prem believed his father was a dry drunk as a result of unresolved intergenerational trauma and social learning from his lineage.

At the age of five, Prem's mother became very sick due to maternal sepsis after childbirth. He recalls collecting healing herbs called *kali bhambol*, boiling them with water, and feeding the liquid to his mother so that she would survive. This was his first traumatic experience. He also missed six months of school due to regional illnesses, including malaria, typhoid, and jaundice. Prem survived the *1947 Partition of India/Pakistan* (Dalrymple, 2015); fortunately, his family was not as significantly impacted given they lived on the India side. Prem recalls witnessing not only the mistreatment of women but also the deaths of Muslims who were fired upon; this gun violence bothered him, as some of his friends were Muslim.

Despite experiencing worrisome illnesses throughout his life, Prem still completed his studies. His grade point average was mediocre due to his poor health, which influenced his father to believe that he was not smart. To prove his father wrong, Prem persisted and eventually completed his bachelor of teaching program. During this time, he had severe attacks of typhoid, became very sick, but was still able to complete his exams. Afterwards, he moved to Delhi and enrolled in a joint master's in psychology and diploma in guidance. In Delhi, Prem was introduced to drinking alcohol and Western colonial ways of living; he became interested in migrating to Canada as he believed he would have more freedom, economic benefits, and academic/professional opportunities.

Upon graduating from his master's program, Prem was hired as a lecturer by his brother, who was the principal of a teacher's training college for women. Prem met his future wife, a student at the college; this was a monumental milestone in his life. Shortly afterwards, he was given immigration status for Canada based on his teaching degree and was hired as a teacher in a small town in Alberta. Before he left for Canada, he informed his future wife that he would return in two years. This left her in complete disbelief as they had planned to get married later that same year. He promised that his stay in Canada would be short-lived and that he would return to India after he accessed and accomplished educational endeavours.

After spending two years of feeling lonely, and adjusting to the climate, culture, people, and cuisine in Canada, Prem returned to India to get married. While living in Canada, he regularly corresponded with his wife by exchanging letters. Soon after their marriage, Prem and his wife returned to Canada but had tremendous marital issues resulting from his wife missing her life and family in India. These were the most traumatic and stressful years of his life. Tragically, while Prem and his wife were finally settling into their life in Canada, Prem's mother passed away from cancer. He was unable to go to her funeral due to having just visited family the summer prior. As an immigrant, he felt powerless and was grieving away from his relatives. Prominent family passings happened over the years; being unable to attend the funerals contributed to his second-guessing mindset around moving to another country. The following year, after his mother died, his first child was born.

During his professional career, Prem encountered different forms of racism while trying to obtain tenure or being promoted to administrative positions within his faculty. These barriers motivated Prem to explore the possibility of returning to India. After the birth of his second child, both he and his wife were offered teaching positions at Punjab University. They moved back to India, but this only lasted four months as both of their children became dehydrated due to the Indian climate. His wife was also pregnant with their third child. There was immense resistance from his older brothers about moving back to Canada, but the decision was obvious. They were fortunate enough to reclaim their previous jobs. Their third child was born shortly after returning to Canada. Six months later; Prem's father died of a severe stroke. Prem was unable to attend his funeral with other family members, and thus grieved alone.

Raising a family in Canada from the late 1960s to 2000 also involved experiencing diverse types of racism, such as microaggressions, and intercultural/interfaith tension. Prem was able to navigate these events and situations to the best of his ability and awareness. He spent most of his weekends hosting cultural events for his children and intergenerational community members. From a surplus, abandoned, and dehydrated village kid of average intelligence, and through sheer willpower, Prem became a mobile, established, professionally active person who moved from rural India to teach at a Canadian university. In his old age, he often regrets his immigrant experiences and believes everything, including his marriage, career, and raising a family, could have easily been accomplished had he stayed in India. He will likely grieve his fractured sense of self and lack of belongingness to both cultures, which all need to be validated on a therapeutic level. Yet considering the historical, political, and current situation in India, he realizes making Canada his home was worthwhile. Does Prem assume he will always grieve?

Isla

Isla is a 40-year-old Latine heterosexual cisgender female. She lives in El Salvador where she was surrounded by gang violence, high crime rates, and overall systemic corruption. Isla grew up in a small town called Arambala south of the Honduran border. She spent most of her childhood and adolescence working at her family's hotel business and caring for her five younger siblings, whom she adored. She inconsistently attended grade school and withdrew after completing grade eight. She had decided to learn how to manage the hotel in hopes of it providing other work opportunities later in life.

At the age of seven years, Isla witnessed members of the *Mara Salvatrucha* gang torture and murder her maternal uncle (Wolf, 2012). Knowing the corruption that exists in El Salvador, one might consider these occurrences part of the culture; however, Isla was deeply affected by this event and carries that trauma with her to present day. She is perpetually reminded of this event if she hears random gun shots at night; when she hears these sounds, she defaults to freeze or fawn trauma responses, has a panic attack, and dissociates from reality until she can centre and ground herself in the present moment. These episodes can last up to one to three hours.

By the time she was 17-year-old, Isla was married off to a man from Perquin, a town north of Arambala. She had only met him once with his devout Roman Catholic parents. Isla's parents coordinated this union, knowing that she needed to focus on the next phase of her life, which meant living with her in-laws and having children. Isla had other aspirations and was planning on opening her business. Isla expressed her vision to her parents, but she felt dismissed and was forced to move away from Arambala and succumb to this involuntary situation.

As a young wife to a husband who was 10 years her senior and in-laws who expected her to cater to the entire extended family, Isla felt abandoned by her parents. She rarely reconnected with them as she was preoccupied with taking care of her husband and his family. She tried to make the most of this situation by having her first child at age 19 and twins at age 21. Two years later, she almost died while giving birth to a stillborn child. This significant loss and overwhelming grief caused added friction to Isla's already tenuous marriage. She questioned whether all the familial expectations caused the stillbirth and if this child could have been saved if she felt more supported by her in-laws. Her husband claimed that this was God's vision for their family and that they were indeed supposed to have only three children.

Isla endured another 10 years of marriage and life with her in-laws. During this time, the overall familial dynamics became progressively worse. Her in-laws started to exclude her from extended family events, and her husband enabled their actions towards Isla. Her husband started using drugs and "working late nights," which eventually translated to Isla learning about the countless extramarital affairs he had over the course of their marriage. Feelings of inadequacy and failure occupied Isla's mind and soul. She redirected her focus towards her children, ensuring that they all became educated and eventually financially independent. She finally confided in her mother about what was happening in her life; shocked and saddened, Isla's mother, with the assistance of her husband and older brother, helped Isla *leave* the marriage with her three children and return to her parents' home in Arambala. By feeling heard and respected by them, Isla was able to forge a renewed relationship with her parents.

It has taken over seven years for Isla to make sense of having frequently second-guessed her choices. She is learning to heal from the range of traumas she encountered over the course of her life. Isla is hoping to work with a culturally responsive and trauma-informed psychotherapist who is well versed in C-PTSD. For the sake of herself and her children, she would like to come to terms with her past traumas and reconnect with her family.

Yin

Yin is a 34-year-old heterosexual cisgender female and second-generation Chinese immigrant. She migrated to the United States at the age of five years with her older brother, parents, and grandparents from a small village called Tai'an. Her family's reasons for migration echo the words of most immigrants: to provide better academic and professional opportunities for their children. Yin's father was a farmer in China, and his entire family helped maintain the farm. Yin's paternal aunt lived abroad in New Jersey and offered to sponsor their family. The immigration process happened very quickly, and within two years, Yin's family landed in Newark, New Jersey. Thankfully, they were able to stay with Yin's paternal aunt until they felt settled enough to live in their own house.

Yin's family barely spoke English; however, they attended English as a Second Language (ESL) classes and other government-funded immigrant settlement programs prior to finding viable employment. Yin's parents worked in different factories before opening a restaurant serving authentic Chinese food. Yin spent her leisure time playing the flute and drawing, which she found relaxing. Her earliest memories of living in the United States included being called racist names and being teased for her homemade clothes. Even though their neighbourhood was culturally diverse, other multicultural students felt that the teachers treated Yin and her brother differently due to their ability to quickly learn lesson plans. This was Yin's first encounter with both the model minority myth and racism.

Yin recalls her parents talking about the 1989 *Tiananmen Square Protests and Massacre* (Sarotte, 2012). Yin's paternal aunt was enrolled in college at the time and was brutally killed during these riots. While their village is five hours away from Beijing, Yin's family continued to be traumatized by this historical two-month event, which led them to consider leaving China. Yin was born only one year before these riots and still feels the effects of these events resounding through her body. Her father has never been the same and feels immense guilt for not protecting his younger sister. Yin's grandparents, who lived with them at the time of migration, never recovered from these events, continue to be in flight mode, and constantly need to be busy all the time.

To add to these horrific events, Yin was sexually assaulted when she was 11-years-old by a close family friend. She was having a playdate at a friend's house when her friend's father cornered her and started inappropriately touching her. Yin bravely told him to stop, but he continued until he heard a door open and then briskly walked away. Yin froze while trying to tell her parents what happened but was unable to articulate the sequence of events. Her parents tried to understand what she was conveying; but, Yin became silent and never spoke of this incident again.

Throughout Yin's schooling, she felt she needed to adhere to the model minority myth. She was often called upon by teachers to assist students that were struggling with their courses. Her teachers deemed her to be hard-working and autonomous in her school work; however, Yin was dealing with her internal struggles and layers of trauma that required processing. She accessed support from her guidance counsellor and was met with microaggressions and dated stereotypes about Chinese people. Yin did not feel heard or seen by her guidance counsellor, who essentially viewed Yin as more of a role model for other disadvantaged students, believing that nothing could possibly be wrong in her life.

Yin spent her twenties debunking myths about her ethnicity. She enrolled in a non-business degree at university and instead chose to study Asian history. She decided that she would like to become a professor and properly educate others about Chinese culture. In winter 2020, at the beginning of the COVID-19 pandemic, while teaching at a university in the United States, Yin was a potential target of an anti-Asian hate crime. She was told to go home or she would be killed. She was aware that this was becoming more commonplace as the host culture was deliberately blaming Asians for the existence of the COVID-19 pandemic. In that moment, Yin knew it was time to finally confront the multiple layers of trauma that she had been suppressing all these years. She was at a point in her life where regardless of what she accomplished, her past was resurfacing and creating racial barriers around her; these obstacles were stagnating her personal and professional development.

References

Blue, A. W., Darou, W. G., & Ruano, C. (2015). Through silence we speak: Approaches to counselling and psychotherapy with Canadian First Nation clients. *Online Readings in Psychology and Culture, 10*(3), 3–42.

Dalrymple, W. (2015, June 22). The great divide: The violent legacy of Indian partition. *The New Yorker*. www.newyorker.com/magazine/2015/06/29/the-great-divide-books-dalrymple

Sarotte, M. E. (2012). China's fear of contagion: Tiananmen Square and the power of the European example. *International Security*, *37*(2), 156–182.

Tesar, A. (2022). Reserves in Nova Scotia. In *The Canadian Encyclopedia*. Retrieved August 19, 2022, from www.thecanadianencyclopedia.ca/en/article/reserves-in-nova-scotia

Winters, M. F. (2020). *Black fatigue: How racism erodes the mind, body, and spirit*. Berrett-Koehler Publishers, Inc.

Wolf, S. (2012). Mara Salvatrucha: The most dangerous street gang in the Americas? *Latin American Politics and Society*, *54*(1), 65–99.

Part 4

Navigating Clinical Implications

Linking Theory to Practice

Introduction

To start, it is fundamental to define psychotherapy and how it is represented in different cultural spheres. Psychotherapy is "any psychological procedure that is aimed at relieving an individual's psychological suffering" (Tseng & Streltzer, 2001, p. 7). The *Ontario Psychotherapy Act* elucidates the practice of psychotherapy as "the assessment and treatment of cognitive, emotional or behavioural disturbances by psychotherapeutic means, delivered through a therapeutic relationship based primarily on verbal or non-verbal communication" (Ontario Psychotherapy Act, 2007 Section 3). Ideally, the objective of one's psychotherapeutic process is for the client(s) to leave with concrete resources and tools that are beneficial in nurturing a positive mindset.

Psychotherapy consists of talk therapy, techniques, collateral sources, interviews, observations, and Western leaning assessments. Although, within a cultural context, this type of information gathering or support may appear too structured. Often BIPOC seeking help or guidance meet with a healer to resolve their presenting concern and ameliorate their mental health. Western or colonial approaches may detract from this collaborative therapeutic rapport, which is needed to foster the safety and trust for clients to consistently engage in the therapeutic process (Audet & Paré, 2017; Paré, 2013).

Collectivist and individualist worldviews are frequently brought forth by my BIPOC clients. As stated in my first book, I remarked:

In working with multicultural populations, individualistic and collectivistic traits require consideration. A clinician should be aware that a dichotomous facet exists between the immediate family and extended family dynamics (Shariff, 2009; Sodhi, 2008). Likewise, as clinicians it is important to discern the family structure and the impact on the family's functioning, whether it is individualistic or collectivistic in nature,

DOI: 10.4324/9781003216568-11

and what family rules, expectations, traditions, and rituals are practices in the household.

(Sodhi, 2017, p. 128)

How can we provide services that encourage BIPOC to access therapy without feeling stigmatized? What might be required is the normalization of seeking help outside of family and community while simultaneously appreciating that there are culturally responsive practitioners available to provide support and guidance. This is a work in progress which commands a collective effort from therapists of diverse intersectional and trauma-informed backgrounds. In due time, hopefully clients will feel empowered to break barriers and intergenerational cycles.

For BIPOC, therapists must consider how each group perceives and accepts mental health, therapy, circle of care involvement, and community to heal from adversity. The stigmatization of mental health continues to be discernable in BIPOC communities and is repeatedly described in physical contexts (Koç & Kafa, 2019; Sodhi, 2017). Individuals may name their mental health issues in somatic terms, such as headaches, stomach problems, and so on due to fear of being judged, alienated, or excluded by family members for discussing their concerns. Some may categorize their mental health issues as a "punishment from God" (Rössler, 2016, p. 1250) or a cultural curse, again deterring themselves from accessing help, although a *safer* form of support is often sought within the cultural/ethnic/racial community.

Similarly, innumerable types of psychotherapy have been present in a multitude of cultures. Buddhists have been practicing psychotherapy for over 2,000 years, primarily to understand and heal from suffering. Monks would essentially *educate* or *counsel* community members to a state of enlightenment and self-awareness which indirectly helped overcome their personal problem(s) (Marma, 2017; Thich, 1999). The Japanese developed *Ikigai*, which demonstrates how one can live a meaningful and purposeful life or a *reason for being*. "Iki" in Japanese denotes "life," and "gai" defines one's value or worth. The Ikigai framework considers elements such as values, possibilities, gifts, and passions and how these facets can influence perspectives about the world, making a difference, and areas of growth (García & Miralles, 2017).

South Asian psychotherapy draws more from balanced mind-body traditions such as Ayurvedic (e.g., meditation, yoga, herbal medicines, custom diets), Hindu, Yogic, Buddhist, and Bhakti (devotional) approaches. Ayurveda, known as "the Science of Life," pays homage to one's "spiritual, mental, and social health" (Behere et al., 2013, p. S310). *Satvavajaya* or psychotherapy addresses three main tenets: replacement of emotions, assurances, and psycho-shock therapy; Satvavajava is fuelled by the set of emotions that make up one's psychopathology (Tripathi, 2012). Again, the focus is on one's overall wellbeing.

Offering exclusively Western psychotherapeutic approaches is yet another "form of continued oppression and colonization, as it does not legitimize the Indigenous cultural view of mental health" (Stewart, 2008, p. 48). Stewart accentuates that Indigenous mental health and healing should include community, cultural identity, holistic approaches, and interdependence that are not rooted in colonial principles (2008). As such, Indigenous healing practices consist of, smudging, drumming ceremonies, the use of herbal medicine, and the medicine wheel which depicts physical, mental, emotional, and spiritual aspects of the individual's life (Ford-Ellis, 2019; Marsh et al., 2015). The medicine wheel is multipurpose and can be used to learn about and heal past relationships with oneself and others as well as to determine one's purpose in life (Rutherford, 2009). Lastly, like decolonized ideologies, the Indigenous concept of two-eyed seeing is an amalgam of traditional Indigenous and Western practices to nurture holistic healing (Marsh et al., 2016). Two-eyed seeing is "a profound guiding principle that encourages self-reflection and emphasizes the transformational capacity of knowledge" (Forbes et al., 2020, p. 2).

In addition to feminist and anti-oppressive therapies, relational cultural theory or therapy espouses treating clients from a socially just angle. Honing in on the therapeutic relationship, therapists cultivate a socially just milieu with the client which serves as a vehicle for comprehending their mental health disparities (Comstock et al., 2008; Jordan, 2017). Relational cultural theory emphasizes that healing occurs through the connection, compassion, and trust that enables clients to feel safe and therapeutically grow (Duffey & Trepal, 2016; Liang, 2022; Rector-Aranda, 2019).

Historically speaking, the cultural/ethnic/racial breakdown of those who attend therapy skews more towards eurocentric individuals than BIPOC (Breslau et al., 2017). Chapter 6 delineates barriers hindering BIPOC from accessing therapy, including cultural stigma associated with therapy, level of engagement, and frequency of appointments. What has repeatedly transpired in my sessions are conversations about the initial challenges of starting the therapeutic process, including "structural racism, racial microaggressions, model-minority stereotypes, and the role that familial and spiritual influences play in seeking help for mental health issues" (Hingwe, 2021, p. 85). Some of my BIPOC clients have expressed that therapy was a much-needed support that required accessing guidance outside of family and community to unlearn and resolve their presenting problem(s). Other BIPOC clients mentioned that their peers had talked openly about their therapeutic experiences and noticed a difference in their self-perception, which thusly encouraged them to try therapy, too.

Factors impacting whether one accesses help are intersectionality, privilege regarding the awareness of systems, and ability to vanquish barriers. I am adamant about mitigating therapeutic withdrawal rates by further reinforcing decolonial approaches with prospective clients during the initial consultation; this shared understanding assures them of being witnessed and valued. Clients have additionally remarked on their self- or assumed stigma associated with seeking help outside of their familial or community systems. Even calling 911 or going to the emergency department comes with the fear of being judged by others: who will see them, or will their employer/immigration find out or have access to the psychiatric (discharge) report? These intrusive thoughts delay BIPOC from acquiring relevant healthcare assistance and guidance. And so, the cycle perpetuates.

Therapeutic Perspective

My therapeutic approach with BIPOC is integrative, eclectic, and intentionally utilizes decolonized methods (Sodhi, 2021; Tuck & Yang, 2012). In the introduction, I mention my leaning towards an *intersectional feminist* framework. Furthermore, my approach is comprised of ethnographic inquiry and postmodernism narrative methods (e.g., co-construction of the client's cultural story). As cited in Seeley (2004), Geertz (1973) states that "ethnography involves modes of observation and inquiry that produce dense, multilayered, and complex accounts of cultures from the perspectives of those who inhabit them" (p. 123). Both methods complement an intersectional feminist approach and lend to a more conversational style of therapy that couples well with psychoeducation on an as-needed basis (Semmler & Williams, 2000).

Given mental health dialogues are being silenced, oral storytelling/history resonates with BIPOC as it is one of "the oldest forms of communication" (Jenkins, 2013, p. 141) that continues to be timely today. For example, in Indigenous healing circles, talking sticks are used so that members who are holding the stick take turns speaking and sharing stories and narratives. This process offers a safe and uninterrupted space to speak and allows for traditions to be carefully passed down to future generations (Baesler, 2019; Baldwin, 1998). In therapy, oral storytelling allows clients to recount what their ancestors have taught and passed down to them and connect their narratives to their descendants. Clients can listen to and reclaim their narratives while therapists gather relevant information (Dennis & Minor, 2019). In keeping with the traditions of oral storytelling, I document minimal notes, capturing global statements that encapsulate the essence of what the client is conveying as well as their affect. Focusing on spoken stories allows for frequent and empathic eye contact, which invites clients to engage in momentous dialogue and share stories that respect and honour ancestral suffering. My efforts are to be more relational and connect with the client during the initial stages of therapy (Hardy, 2018). I am mindful about not "conducting" an interview (in the form of Western assessment and evaluation) but to have purposeful therapeutic conversation. I meet the client where they are at, incorporate Eastern therapeutic modalities, avoid diagnostic labelling/pathologizing, explore unwelcomed systems, and pose reflective questions.

My BIPOC clients have taught me that attendance can be erratic; there may be inconsistency or pauses during therapy. Select clients will commit to therapy for the long haul, while other clients withdraw or prematurely terminate from the process around the sixth session benchmark. This might occur after sharing a difficult part of their life, which could cause regret and/or embarrassment. My intention is to ensure that there is continuity of care, validation, and walking alongside the client throughout their complete therapeutic process. To enhance this initiative, I use familiar language to build safety and trust with the client and messaging that hinders the activation of their nervous system (Ibaraki & Hall, 2014). I try to utilize as much common language with my clients to help diminish feelings of shame/guilt as well as offer a more community atmosphere. Therapeutic protocols – especially limits to confidentiality and boundaries with family – are reinforced throughout the entire process. This way of being has engendered overwhelmingly positive feedback from clients due to feeling culturally respected.

The next three chapters outline decolonized psychotherapeutic practices, introduce inclusion and healing therapy (IHT), and analyze and implement IHT utilizing narratives from Part 3.

References

Audet, C., & Paré, D. (Eds.). (2017). *Social justice and counselling: Discourse in practice*. Routledge.

Baesler, E. J. (2019). From talking stick to listening stick: A variation on an ancient practice. *Listening Education, 9*(2), 17–34.

Baldwin, C. (1998). *Calling the circle: The first and future culture*. Bantam.

Behere, P. B., Das, A., Yadav, R., & Behere, A. P. (2013). Ayurvedic concepts related to psychotherapy. *Indian Journal of Psychiatry, 55*(Suppl 2), S310–S314.

Breslau, J., Cefalu, M., Wong, E. C., Burnam, M. A., Hunter, G. P., Florez, K. R., & Collins, R. L. (2017). Racial/ethnic differences in perception of need for mental health treatment in a US national sample. *Social Psychiatry and Psychiatric Epidemiology, 52*(8), 929–937.

Comstock, D. L., Hammer, T. R., Strentzch, J., Cannon, K., Parsons, J., & Salazar II, G. (2008). Relational-cultural theory: A framework for bridging relational, multicultural, and social justice competencies. *Journal of Counselling and Development, 86*(3), 279–287.

Dennis, M., & Minor, M. (2019). Healing through storytelling: Indigenising social work with stories. *The British Journal of Social Work, 49*(6), 1472–1490.

Duffey, T., & Trepal, H. (2016). Introduction to the special section on relational-cultural theory. *Journal of Counseling and Development, 94*(4), 379–382.

Forbes, A., Ritchie, S. D., Walker, J., & Young, N. L. (2020). Applications of two-eyed seeing in primary research focused on Indigenous health: A scoping review. *International Journal of Qualitative Methods, 19*, 1–18.

Ford-Ellis, A. G. (2019). How is the medicine wheel considered in therapeutic practice? *Journal of Concurrent Disorders, 1*(3), 78–93.

García, H., & Miralles, F. (2017). *IKIGAI: The Japanese secret to living a long and happy life.* Penguin Life.

Geertz, C. (1973). *The interpretation of cultures.* Basic Books.

Hardy, K. V. (2018). The self of the therapist in epistemological context: A multicultural relational perspective. *Journal of Family Psychotherapy, 29*(1), 17–29.

Hingwe, S. (2021). Mental health considerations for Black, Indigenous, and People of Color: Trends, barriers, and recommendations for collegiate mental health. *College Psychiatry, 1*, 85–96.

Ibaraki, A. Y., & Hall, G. C. N. (2014). The components of cultural match in psychotherapy. *Journal of Social and Clinical Psychology, 33*(10), 936–953.

Jenkins, S. (2013). Counselling and storytelling: How did we get here? *Psychotherapy and Politics International, 11*(2), 140–151.

Jordan, J. V. (2017). Relational-cultural theory: The power of connection to transform our lives. *Journal of Humanistic Counseling, 56*(3), 228–243.

Koç, V., & Kafa, G. (2019). Cross-cultural research on psychotherapy: The need for a change. *Journal of Cross-Cultural Psychology, 50*(1), 100–115.

Liang, C. T. H. (2022). An intersectional perspective on relational-cultural theory: Commentary on Di Bianca and Mahalik. *The American Psychologist, 77*(3), 336–337.

Marma, A. (2017). Counseling and its importance: A Buddhist perspective. *Journal of the International Association of Buddhist Universities, 7*(1), 29–41.

Marsh, T. N., Coholic, D., Cote-Meek, S., & Najavits, L. M. (2015). Blending Aboriginal and western healing methods to treat intergenerational trauma with substance use disorder in Aboriginal peoples who live in Northeastern Ontario, Canada. *Harm Reduction Journal, 12*(14), 1–12.

Marsh, T. N., Cote-Meek, S., Young, N. L., Najavits, L. M., & Toulouse, P. (2016). Indigenous healing and seeking safety: A blended implementation project for intergenerational trauma and substance use disorders. *International Indigenous Policy Journal, 7*(2), 1–35.

Ontario Psychotherapy Act. (2007). Retrieved June 6, 2022, from www.ontario.ca/laws/statute/07p10#ys3

Paré, D. A. (2013). *The practice of collaborative counselling and psychotherapy: Developing skills in culturally mindful helping.* Sage Publications.

Rector-Aranda, A. (2019). Critically compassionate intellectualism in teacher education: The contributions of relational-cultural theory. *Journal of Teacher Education, 70*(4), 388–400.

Rössler, W. (2016). The stigma of mental disorders: A millennia-long history of social exclusion and prejudices. *EMBO Reports, 17*(9), 1250–1253.

Rutherford, L. (2009) A shamanic approach to psychotherapy. *Self & Society, 37*(1), 10–17.

Seeley, K. M. (2004). Short-term intercultural psychotherapy: Ethnographic inquiry. *Social Work, 49*(1), 121–130.

Semmler, P. L., & Williams, C. B. (2000). Narrative therapy: A storied context for multicultural counseling. *Journal of Multicultural Counseling & Development*, 28(1), 51–60.

Shariff, A. (2009). Ethnic identity and parenting stress in South Asian families: Implications for culturally sensitive counselling. *Canadian Journal of Counselling*, 43(1), 35–46.

Sodhi, P. K. (2008). Bicultural identity formation of second-generation Indo-Canadians. *Canadian Ethnic Studies*, 40(2), 187–199.

Sodhi, P. K. (2017). *Exploring immigrant and sexual minority mental health: Reconsidering multiculturalism*. Routledge.

Sodhi, P. K. (2021). Decolonizing psychotherapeutic practices for BIPOC clients. Webinar hosted by the *Canadian Counselling and Psychotherapy Association*, October 27, 2021.

Stewart, S. (2008). Promoting Indigenous mental health: Cultural perspectives on healing from Native counsellors in Canada. *International Journal of Health Promotion and Education*, 46(2), 49–56.

Thich, N. H. (1999). *The heart of the Buddha' teaching: Transforming suffering into peace, joy, and liberation*. Broadway Books.

Tripathi, J. S. (2012). Dimensions of sattvavajaya chikitsa (ayurvedic-psychotherapy) and their clinical applications. *Annals of Ayurvedic Medicine*, 1, 31–38.

Tseng, W.-S., & Streltzer, J. (Eds.). (2001). *Culture and psychotherapy: A guide to clinical practice*. American Psychiatric Publishing, Inc.

Tuck, E., & Yang, W. K. (2012). Decolonization is not a metaphor. *Decolonization: Indigeneity, Education & Society*, 1(1), 1–40.

Chapter 7

Decolonizing Mental Health Practices

This chapter delineates decolonized mental health practices; establishing a safe therapeutic rapport with BIPOC; Eastern, Western, and ethical space considerations; and closes with a practical framework highlighting these perspectives.

What Are Decolonized Mental Health Practices?

Decolonizing one's thinking involves liberation from a colonized mindset; it is a process of deconditioning, focussing, and exploring how unresolved layers of trauma, racism, capitalism, and other forms of oppression have systemically impacted one's own mental health. Decolonization of mental health practices includes using lived experience and interventions such as ancestral work, intergenerational trauma, and increasing connecting; taking such steps allows "communities to decide what is considered suffering, rather than having the system decide for them" (Khúc as referenced in Zapata, 2020; Sodhi, 2021). Furthermore, Dr. Jennifer Mullan, founder of *Decolonizing Therapy*, affirms:

> we do a lot of ancestral work, a lot of intergenerational trauma work, dealing with rage as a function and a normal understanding system of living in a world that continues to oppress us and not provide many of us with what we need.

Therefore, "decolonization is not a metaphor and trying to be better mental health advocates is not going to be enough. Being culturally competent, in my humble, loving opinion, is not enough" (Zapata, 2020).

Instead, practitioners must be attentive to how colonization along with white supremacy, capitalism, and patriarchy have negatively influenced the current BIPOC mindset. Given our polarized sociopolitical climate, it is crucial to integrate decolonized or Indigenized mental health practices within our work with BIPOC clients by shifting from individualist,

DOI: 10.4324/9781003216568-12

Western psychology/approaches to more collectivist, Eastern/inclusive practices (Bhargava et al., 2016). Western psychotherapeutic approaches are not a "one-size-fits-all" phenomena. To better support BIPOC, we need to decolonize the *Diagnostic and Statistical Manual of Mental Disorders* (DSM-5), accessing help, attachment styles, inner child work, and trauma care so that increased awareness, fewer colonial repercussions, and anti-oppressive frameworks are represented in our practice with BIPOC clients. Some focus on neurobiology certainly has a place in anti-racist practice. However, by incorporating elements of neurobiology while omitting cultural differences, the *DSM-5* revives and fortifies colonialism in current psychotherapy practice (Bredström, 2019).

We are evolving as mental health professionals, yet there is still plenty of room for growth and awareness around implementing decolonized practices. Listed are suggestions pertinent to decolonizing one's own therapeutic practice:

- Look beyond symptomology and explore the origins of clients' potential mental health conditions, particularly if there is somatization involved. In Western psychology there is more emphasis on mental health symptoms, whereas decolonized approaches delve into the client's narrative and systemic causes (Oluo, 2018).
- Manifest a trauma-informed and anti-racist worldview, explore systemic implications, and provide therapy utilizing a comprehensive intersectional framework (Crenshaw, 1991).
- Reword Western assessments such as the PCL-5 (post-traumatic checklist) to include simpler and culturally responsive language.
- Work from an integrated community care perspective; nurture safe connections supported by equitable and intentional actions.
- Lean into one's intersectionality and provide therapy grounded in collectivist theoretical orientations and collective healing.
- Offer accessible services by having a sliding scale fee and alternative session locations/modalities.
- Discontinue labelling clients with Western psychological diagnoses as they may be incongruent with what the client is somatically experiencing.
- Use family interviews and recognize the cultural differences and nuances that are fundamental in learning more about an individual's background and history.

By adhering to decolonizing mental health practices, therapists focus on normalizing therapy in BIPOC families and communities and understanding and respecting the client's capacity to achieve therapeutic aspirations and tasks.

Therapeutic Rapport

To reiterate, developing a safe and trusting therapeutic alliance is essential for BIPOC to feel seen, heard, and valued in the therapeutic space. Assessing therapeutic progress can be considered more colonial and eurocentric in nature. If we invest and nurture the therapeutic dynamic, progress will follow. If we hyperfocus on progress and achieving benchmarks, we may paradoxically undermine progress by neglecting the therapeutic alliance; therefore, I consciously focus on the process versus the outcome in my work. We can strengthen the therapeutic rapport by decentring hierarchal and power differentials.

By prioritizing rapport, therapists are promoting access and equity to therapy; this may be due to therapists understanding the client's overall intersectionality and worldviews, thus fostering the client's sense of belonging and connection to a community with parallel commonalities. Modelling open and respectful dialogue about systematic oppression bolsters trust within the therapeutic rapport (Meyer & Zane, 2013). Additionally, fostering therapeutic attunement where the therapist is in sync with the client's communication, needs, and expectations strengthens the therapeutic alliance. As a former student once said, "Clients vote with their feet"; that is, they attend, benefit, and return to therapy sessions based on their gratification with the therapeutic progress.

There is a conspicuous lack of empirical research about client-counsellor matching or cultural/ethnic/race related matching (Merali, 1999; Meyer & Zane, 2013) and whether such alignment is necessary for clients to unequivocally engage in the therapeutic process. We cannot assume that intersectional overlap ensures therapeutic compatibility, increased retention rates, or optimal therapeutic outcomes (Ertl et al., 2019). Some clients may feel uncomfortable self-disclosing to a therapist who is of the same cultural/ethnic/racial background due to confidentiality concerns; however, some may perceive the opposite, which highlights cultural humility (Foronda et al., 2016; Hook et al., 2017). Matching backgrounds could add to the shift from culturally competent to cultural humility practices, specifically, self-awareness, demonstrating an egalitarian therapeutic milieu, and working in solidarity with other like-minded individuals (Lekas et al., 2020; Mollen & Ridley, 2021; Tervalon & Murray-García, 1998).

Ratts et al. (2015) offer insight in their *Multicultural and Social Justice Counseling Competencies* (MSJCC) model. This model illustrates the necessity of accentuating intersectional identities between the counsellor and client. The MSJCC model is an extension of work by Sue et al. (1992), which imparts awareness about multicultural counselling competencies (MCC). The MSJCC model suggests that systems of oppression, power, and privilege can be further examined and discussed within the therapeutic dynamic and combines both collectivist and individualist worldviews.

The MSJCC model consists of four quadrants: (1) privileged counsellor – marginalized client, (2) privileged counsellor – privileged client, (3) marginalized counsellor – privileged client, and (4) marginalized counsellor – marginalized client (Ratts et al., 2015, 2016), demonstrating the variety of statuses, systemic combinations, and interactions between the client and counsellor. It is further divided into four domains: (1) counsellor self-awareness, (2) client worldview, (3) counselling relationship, (4) counselling and advocacy interventions. These domains depict the various layers of multicultural and social justice competence between the counsellor and client. Cultural competencies are exterior to the outer ring of the model and include attitudes and beliefs, knowledge, skills, and actions. These cultural competencies remain imperative for the counsellor to follow alongside cultural humility and cultural responsiveness (Hook et al., 2017).

Eastern, Western, and Ethical Space Considerations

Appreciating the intersection between Eastern and Western ideologies support decolonized treatment planning and long-term therapy to BIPOC clients (Forbes et al., 2020). As mentioned in Figure 7.1, Eastern and Western perspectives each offer their own rendition of therapy. Eastern ideologies integrates familial and community support, collective and multicultural healing traditions, and anti-oppressive psychotherapeutic strategies; in contrast, Western ideologies subscribe to autonomously working towards therapeutic intentions, eurocentric and colonial techniques, and rigidity surrounding session modality and fee schedule. Interestingly, the overlap between both systems suggests leveraging collaboration, culturally responsive circle of care, no *DSM-5* diagnoses or labels, and meeting the client where they are at in the therapeutic process.

Donald (2009) asserts that due to the historical oppression within North America, it is necessary to "organize" and "separate" people "according to race, culture, and civilization" (p. 4). This reframe essentially pays homage to and respects the experiences of different oppressed groups and allows for individuals to feel less affected by colonialism. The purpose of this separation is not to racially segregate in a way that supports white supremacy but instead to offer the support that marginalized groups need to overturn white supremacy. Donald contends "that decolonization in a Canadian context can only occur when Aboriginal peoples and Canadians face each other across historic divides, deconstruct their shared past, and engage critically with the realization that their present and future is similarly tied together" (p. 5). Lacerda-Vandenborn refers to this as a "third space," which is the intersection between Western and Indigenous perceptions and is integral to decolonizing mental health practices (Zapata, 2020).

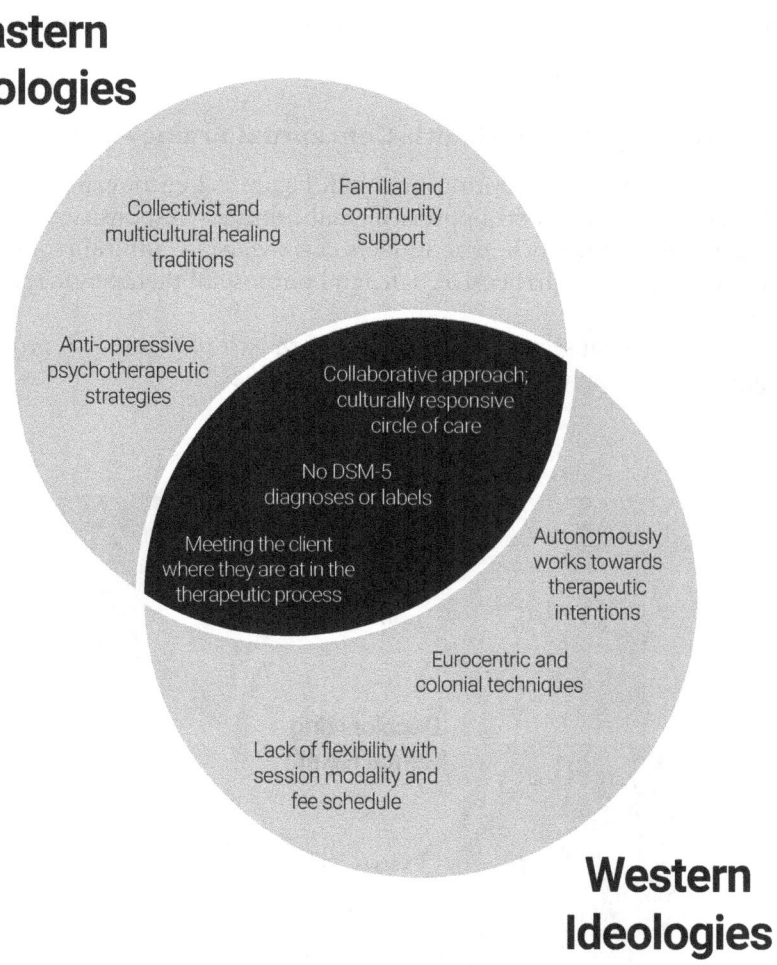

Eastern Ideologies

Collectivist and multicultural healing traditions

Familial and community support

Anti-oppressive psychotherapeutic strategies

Collaborative approach; culturally responsive circle of care

No DSM-5 diagnoses or labels

Meeting the client where they are at in the therapeutic process

Autonomously works towards therapeutic intentions

Eurocentric and colonial techniques

Lack of flexibility with session modality and fee schedule

Western Ideologies

Figure 7.1 Eastern and Western therapeutic ideologies

Congruently, Ermine (2007) proposes that an "ethical space is formed when two societies, with disparate worldviews, are poised to engage each other" (p. 193). Engagement fosters open and safe conversation, active listening, and relationship building between the two systems (Laurila, 2019). In the real world, this would consist of individuals meeting in person to discuss ethical and spiritual topics that impact various levels of civilization (Ermine, 2007). Eventually, by investing in an ethical space, meaningful, shared, and respectful exchanges will occur and subsequently decentre positions of power, stereotypes, and oppressive systems.

Decolonizing Mental Health Conceptual Framework

Keeping these considerations in mind, Figure 7.2 encompasses trauma-informed, anti-racist, anti-oppressive, and culturally responsive principles. By using this framework, practitioners can engage in cultural inquiry and thus cultivate a comprehensive, safe, and purposeful therapeutic space for their BIPOC clients.

The subsequent sections elaborate on each part of Figure 7.2, providing suggestions to apply these ideologies into practice.

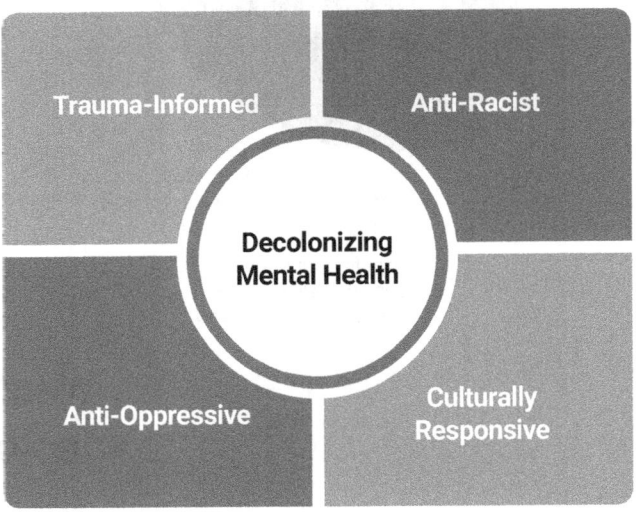

Figure 7.2 Decolonizing mental health

Trauma-Informed

- Remain aware of the client's background or past, create a safe space, and maintain safety by not retraumatizing the client. Explore nuances associated with offering culturally responsive and applicable trauma interventions.
- Discuss how trauma is stored in the body; explore this via somatic experiencing, polyvagal theory, or psychoeducation about trauma and the brain (Dana, 2021; Levine, 1997; Perry & Winfrey, 2021).

- Address how unjust systems of power contribute to suffering (by means of disconnection), patriarchal boundaries, and oppression-related trauma (Maté & Maté, 2022).
- Cultivate a brave and compassionate space for BIPOC clients to share their traumatic experiences and beliefs about feeling oppressed, attacked, and targeted by ongoing white supremacist acts of violence.
- Unpack and contextualize coming from a culture of silence, being silenced, trauma responses, and intrusive trauma-related thoughts about guilt, shame, and blame.
- Name emotions, consider lived experience, and explore how clients manifest, perpetuate, internalize, and heal from various forms of trauma (e.g., colonial trauma, cultural trauma, developmental trauma, intersectional trauma, post-traumatic stress disorder (PTSD)/complex post-traumatic stress disorder (C-PTSD), migratory trauma, systemic trauma, collective trauma, racial trauma, and intergenerational trauma).
- Parse how traumatic stress is somaticized for each client and how it affects their nervous system and compromises their mental health (Dana, 2018; Maté, 2004; Porges, 2011).

Anti-Racist

- Define systemic factors that have enabled the patriarchy, imperialism, and eurocentricity.
- Explore messages entrenched in systemic racism that result in clients feeling "othered" by members from the host culture/country.
- Unlearn and reframe colonial and racist values, responses, and expectations.
- Identify the impact of racial stereotypes, discrimination, gaslighting, and microaggressions (Sue & Sue, 2019).
- Assist clients navigate covert and overt racism to prevent internalized racism (David et al., 2019; Pyke, 2010).
- Encourage clients to regain pride regarding their cultural/ethnic/racial identity and teach others about the importance of being a productive ally (Akbar, 2020).

Anti-Oppressive

- Dismantle systems of power, privilege, and oppression including racism, classism, colonialism, ableism, sexism, heterosexism, and homophobia (Freire, 1970).
- Critically examine systemic biases and clinical barriers, break historical cycles, and foster resilience in our clients.
- Eradicate stigma associated with help seeking and offer more accessible mental health services.

- Understand what is embedded in systemic oppression and how this is internalized by BIPOC clients.
- Be reminded of our ancestors' powerful lived experience and stories of perseverance.

Culturally Responsive

- Engage in cultural humility (Hook et al., 2016); be culturally curious, self-reflective, and learn from our clients, who are the experts of their narratives.
- Strengthen the learner-expert dichotomy, honour the client as both the learner and the expert, and emphasize the importance of being culturally curious and engaged. There is however a fine line between the therapist becoming a learner of their narrative and learning about their culture. Therapists need to be informed enough about world history and politics to preclude clients from educating practitioners.
- Inspire collaborative therapeutic dialogue and conversation with a purpose (Paré, 2013).
- Recognize the importance of speaking and understanding the same language; learn to sit with the client who is experiencing collective trauma. Be a part of it.
- Silence colonialism and eurocentric therapeutic approaches and replace them with more Eastern and inclusive practices.
- Appreciate the significance of staying current in our language and messaging while working with BIPOC clients.
- Outline the importance of continuous community learning as a safe and allied process.
- Attend trainings and cultural events (e.g., National Indigenous Peoples Day, Chinese New Year, Eid, Juneteenth, Diwali) that exist within BIPOC communities.

Holding space for BIPOC is comprised of cultural empathy, genuineness, congruence, compassion, unconditional positive regard, and supporting clients in silence or pausing during sessions until they are ready to discuss issues. Holding space in this way complements a decolonized therapeutic style. Sustaining therapy with BIPOC can be challenging due to the previously mentioned clinical barriers placed upon them, hence the importance of a safe therapeutic environment.

Cultivating a Safe BIPOC Space

Inspired by Ibram Kendi's chapter on *Space*, I reflected upon how to develop a safe BIPOC space (Kendi, 2019). In his book, Kendi alludes to creating a sustainable space by endorsing literature curated by BIPOC, further representing BIPOC educators in academia, Indigenizing curricula, weaving together Western and Eastern philosophies, invoking cultural humility and inclusivity, using anti-oppressive and anti-racist psychotherapeutic frameworks, and decolonizing therapy. Ideally, such a space would support BIPOC to be completely immersed and esteemed in all aspects of their intersectionality.

By creating safety in therapy, we are encouraging BIPOC to populate diverse spaces, have their voices heard, speak with confidence, be proud of their ancestry, create safe cultural spaces within work and academic milieus, and have faith in their abilities. BIPOC showing up authentically is necessary to decolonization. It can be jarring for BIPOC to consistently present in this manner; however, using oneself representatively is essential to educating others about the intersectional layers of intergenerational trauma and oppression that have affected BIPOC lineage. By being true to themselves, and demonstrating patience with the process, BIPOC and white individuals alike will learn about the repercussions of colonization and white supremacy from BIPOC lived experience.

The next chapter introduces inclusion and healing therapy (IHT), a theoretical framework specifically designed for BIPOC communities.

References

Akbar, M. (2020). *Beyond ally: The pursuit to racial justice*. Publish Your Purpose Press.

Bhargava, R., Kumar, N., & Gupta, A. (2016). Indian perspective on psychotherapy: Cultural issues. *Journal of Contemporary Psychotherapy, 47*, 95–103.

Bredström, A. (2019). Culture and context in mental health diagnosing: Scrutinizing the DSM-5 revision. *Journal of Medical Humanities, 40*, 347–363.

Crenshaw, K. (1991). Mapping the margins: Intersectionality, identity politics, and violence against women of color. *Stanford Law Review, 43*(6), 1241–1299.

Dana, D. (2018). *The polyvagal theory in therapy: Engaging the rhythm of regulation*. W.W. Norton.

Dana, D. (2021). *Anchored: How to befriend your nervous system using polyvagal theory*. Sound True.

David, E. J. R., Schroeder, T. M., & Fernandez, J. (2019). Internalized racism: A systematic review of the psychological literature on racism's most insidious consequence. *Journal of Social Issues, 75*(4), 1057–1086.

Donald, D. (2009). Forts, curriculum, and Indigenous Métissage: Imagining decolonization of Aboriginal-Canadian relations in educational contexts. *First Nations Perspectives, 2*(1), 1–24

Ermine, W. (2007). The ethical space of engagement. *Indigenous Law Journal, 6*(1), 193–203.

Ertl, M. M., Mann-Saumier, M., Martin, R. A., Graves, D. F., & Altarriba, J. (2019). The impossibility of client-therapist "match": Implications and future directions for multicultural competency. *Journal of Mental Health Counseling, 41*(4), 312–326.

Forbes, A., Ritchie, S. D., Walker, J., & Young, N. L. (2020). Applications of two-eyed seeing in primary research focused on Indigenous health: A scoping review. *International Journal of Qualitative Methods*, *19*, 1–18.

Foronda, C., Baptiste, D. L., Reinholdt, M. M., & Ousman, K. (2016). Cultural humility: A concept analysis. *Journal of Transcultural Nursing*, *27*(3), 210–217.

Freire, P. (1970). *Pedagogy of the oppressed*. Continuum International.

Hook, J. N., Don, D., Owen, J., & DeBlaere, C. (2017). *Cultural humility: Engaging diverse identities in therapy* (pp. 43–64). American Psychological Association.

Hook, J. N., Farrell, J. E., Davis, D. E., DeBlaere, C., Van Tongeren, D. R., & Utsey, S. O. (2016). Cultural humility and racial microaggressions in counseling. *Journal of Counseling Psychology*, *63*, 269–277.

Kendi, I. X. (2019). *How to be an antiracist*. One World.

Laurila, K. (2019). *Reconciliation: Facilitating ethical space between Indigenous women and girls of a drum circle and white, settler men of a police chorus* [Theses and dissertations (Comprehensive)], 2114. https://scholars.wlu.ca/etd/2114

Lekas, H.-M., Pahl, K., & Fuller Lewis, C. (2020). Rethinking cultural competence: Shifting to cultural humility. *Health Services Insights*, 1–4.

Levine, P. A. (1997). *Waking the tiger: Healing trauma*. North Atlantic Books.

Maté, G. (2004). *When the body says no: The cost of hidden stress*. Vintage Canada.

Maté, G., & Maté, D. (2022). *The myth of normal: Trauma, illness, and healing in a toxic culture*. Knopf Canada.

Merali, N. (1999). Resolution of value conflicts in multicultural counselling. *Canadian Journal of Counselling*, *33*(1), 28–36.

Meyer, O. L., & Zane, N. (2013). The influence of race and ethnicity in clients' experiences of mental health treatment. *Journal of Community Psychology*, *41*(7), 884–901.

Mollen, D., & Ridley, C. R. (2021). Rethinking multicultural counseling competence: An introduction to the major contribution. *The Counseling Psychologist*, *49*(4), 490–503.

Oluo, I. (2018). *So you want to talk about race*. Seal Press.

Paré, D. A. (2013). *The practice of collaborative counselling and psychotherapy: Developing skills in culturally mindful helping*. SAGE Publications.

Perry, B., & Winfrey, O. (2021). *What happened to you?* Flatiron Books.

Porges, S. W. (2011). *The polyvagal theory: Neurophysiological foundations of emotions, attachment, communication, and self-regulation*. W.W. Norton & Co.

Pyke, K. D. (2010). What is internalized racial oppression and why don't we study it? Acknowledging racism's hidden injuries. *Sociological Perspectives*, *53*, 551–572.

Ratts, M. J., Singh, A. A., Nassar-McMillan, S., Butler, S. K., & McCullough, J. R. (2015). *Multicultural and social justice counseling competencies*. Retrieved July 5, 2022, from www.counseling. org/docs/default-source/competencies/multicultural-and-social-justice-counseling-competencies.pdf?sfvrsn=20

Ratts, M. J., Singh, A. A., Nassar-McMillan, S., Butler, S. K., & McCullough, J. R. (2016). Multicultural and social justice counseling competencies: Guidelines for the counseling profession. *Journal of Multicultural Counseling and Development*, *44*, 28–48.

Sodhi, P. K. (2021). Decolonizing psychotherapeutic practices for BIPOC clients. Webinar hosted by the *Canadian Counselling and Psychotherapy Association*, October 27, 2021.

Sue, D. W., Arredondo, P., & McDavis, R. J. (1992). Multicultural counseling competencies and standards: A call to the profession. *Journal of Multicultural Counseling and Development*, 20(2), 64–88.

Sue, D. W., & Sue, D. (2019). *Counseling the culturally diverse: Theory and practice* (8th ed.). John Wiley & Sons, Inc.

Tervalon, M., & Murray-García, J. (1998). Cultural humility versus cultural competence: A critical distinction in defining physician training outcomes in multicultural education. *Journal of Healthcare for the Poor and Underserved*, 9, 117–125.

Zapata, K. (2020, February 27). *Decolonizing mental health: The importance of an oppression-focused mental health system Calgary Journal.* https://calgaryjournal.ca/more/calgaryvoices/4982-decolonizing-mental-health-the-importance-of-an-oppression-focused-mental-health-system.html/

Chapter 8

Inclusion and Healing Therapy

This chapter amalgamates content from all preceding chapters of this book and introduces a framework and therapeutic approach specifically for all BIPOC who have been subjected to systemic oppression and untold forms of trauma. I developed this framework to support clients in healing from unresolved trauma and feeling more seen within our culturally oppressive society.

Supporting the Client

Therapy sessions should not begin with BIPOC clients providing psychoeducation about their cultural values, beliefs, and traditions; instead, the therapist should be listening to the client's narrative. As a professor, I educate counselling psychology students about finding a balance between being cultural curious versus clients educating the therapist (Sodhi, 2017). A culturally responsive therapist should:

- Hold space
- Empower and introduce agency
- Validate and provide affirmations
- Help regulate and sit with the client and their emotions; name/label the experience
- Be present with the client but not enmeshed in their emotions
- Acknowledge how far the client has progressed by focusing on their strengths and highlighting their growth
- Foster mobilization, active listening, compassion, and unconditional positive regard
- Explore therapist countertransference
- Recognize one's own intersectionality and check in with one's privileges, biases, and prejudices

DOI: 10.4324/9781003216568-13

As part of my existing professional development, I have the honour of supervising novice therapists who have chosen to start a private therapeutic practice. I appreciate the mutual learning and work with these individuals, particularly conversations about the role of the therapist. Based on Jeffrey Kottler's research, therapists do not simply provide therapeutic techniques and interventions; we as therapists need to demonstrate our human side and be authentic and genuine with our actions (Kottler, 2022). It is our responsibility as professionals to identify the pedigree and versatility of theoretical approaches instead of adhering to one therapeutic orientation. There is value in fitting pieces together and keeping one's therapeutic style integrative and current. We are here to guide our clients as experts in our field and not control their involvement in their therapeutic journey.

In another conversation with a current supervisee, we deliberated on the relational nature of narrative therapy and its defocusing of the individual. We talked about narrative therapy as an approach to unpacking white supremacy, the patriarchy, and colonialism; educating others about the supervisee's background/intersectionality; and interrupting the perpetuation of dominant norms and stereotypes. My supervisee shared how he proceeds with the initial stages of therapeutic rapport building and how he breaks down barriers and power dynamics with clients by being implicit at the beginning of treatment; offering a comprehensive informed consent document; recognizing the client as the expert of their narrative; using a culturally responsive framework; learning, teaching, and educating in therapy; utilizing creative questions; and locating strategies to reauthor the narrative. These efforts augment the therapeutic alliance and allow clients to be a part of a safe and collective process.

As therapists, being intentional by asking therapeutic questions to generate meaningful dialogue; working in an egalitarian collaborative space; shifting from therapeutic content to process, or from process to therapeutic outcome; trusting the process; remaining forward facing and building upon progress/rapport, but also staying reflective about the past; tapping into resources (internal and external); normalizing feelings of pain, suffering, and/or disconnection; observing and listening to clients' voices and emotions; and understanding the client's capacity to achieve therapeutic aspirations and tasks makes our work in this field more trauma-informed and inclusive.

Often, BIPOC clients show up (performative) and believe they need therapy; however, they may not be ready to participate (productive) in the therapeutic process or complete the work (e.g., reflections, application of interventions) between sessions. Referring to the resistance, reluctance, and readiness spectrum noted in Chapter 1, I invite clients to explore barriers preventing them from either starting or continuing therapy. Therapists should not work harder than the client. Discussing these barriers from an adversarial standpoint could lead to premature termination of therapy or fear of being judged for sharing reservations for attending therapy. It is often mentioned and reinforced that therapeutic rapport is a mutual venture in which work will be conducted in a united manner. This will ensure that there is therapeutic flow and growth.

The next section acquaints the reader with dynamic aspects of inclusion and healing therapy.

Inclusion and Healing Therapy Framework

Central to creating a culturally responsive trauma-informed theoretical orientation is the decolonization of Western frameworks; these frameworks enable BIPOC to envision themselves participating in mutual therapeutic dialogue. Such decolonization involves identifying and revamping existing oppressive therapeutic approaches and reinstating them with language that is representative and resonates with BIPOC communities (Seeley, 2004). Over the last 25+ years of my career, I have been gradually *infusing* culture and *decolonizing* my therapeutic and teaching methods. I am increasingly aware of my privilege and South Asian ancestry, which have worked to my advantage as I frequently draw from lived experience to decentre Western foundations and replace them with more Eastern wisdom.

The lack of decolonized therapeutic approaches available for BIPOC motivated me to develop an anti-oppressive framework that delineates how clients can understand the impact of internalized oppression and trauma, and therefore grieve and heal from these events. The underpinning tenets of inclusion and healing therapy (IHT) are trauma-informed, anti-racist, anti-oppressive culturally responsive constructs that harness a client's ability to process and actualize a sense of belonging and therefore participate in lifelong healing. Recent third wave cognitive behavioural therapy (CBT) orientations, such as acceptance and commitment therapy (ACT) (Harris, 2008) and culturally adapted CBT (Naeem et al., 2021) demarcate the significance of incorporating decolonized elements (e.g., non-pathologizing clients, exploring intergenerational aspects of suffering, social justice ideologies) within their method, though they lack both the attention to intersectionality and the accessible language that are key to reaching BIPOC.

The *Inclusion and Healing* framework (Figure 8.1) is built upon the *Decolonized Mental Health* framework (see Figure 7.2) to support clients to a place of (radical) acceptance and healing. Clients encounter diverse complexities as they navigate systemic inequalities and barriers, which require a culturally respectful and affirming foundation. This foundation could include family and community considerations that originate from collectivist ideologies. Based on my practice, members of BIPOC communities affirmed experiences (i.e., inequalities and barriers) related to migratory hardships, capitalism, white supremacy, intergenerational trauma, systemic racism and hate crimes, the patriarchy, a lack of identity and sense of belonging, and colonial oppression. Derived from this intel, I have acquired a knowledge base that has led to the evolution of this timely theoretical orientation. The name of this framework summarizes elements of inclusion and healing via a trauma-informed lens. There are different perceptions of trauma-informed care; still, the main premise of trauma-informed care is to support the prevention of retraumatization/re-experiencing while maintaining the safety and stabilization of the client throughout the therapeutic endeavour. Within IHT:

> Inclusion is a dynamic state of operating in which diversity is leveraged to create a fair, healthy, and high-performing organization or community. An inclusive environment ensures equitable access to resources and opportunities for all. It also enables individuals and groups to feel safe, respected, engaged, motivated, and valued for who they are and for their contributions toward organizational and societal goals.
>
> (O'Mara & Richter, 2017, p. 1)

Healing is "achieving or acquiring wholeness as a person" (Egnew, 2005, p. 257). Correspondingly, it is "the process of bringing together aspects of one's self, body-mind-spirit, at deeper levels of inner knowing, leading toward integration and balance with each aspect having equal importance and value" (Dossey & Keegan, 2009, p. 48). Using a cultural lens, healing may include attending to grief, loss, and suffering to foster personal growth and awareness. Some clients may appear to engage in healing but are actually partaking in spiritual bypassing, whereby spirituality becomes a mechanism to circumvent discomfort or unpleasant emotions instead of processing them (Motiño et al., 2021; Trungpa, 2010).

The ethos of IHT is to overcome and process trauma and is thus grounded in naming wounds, retrospective healing, self-compassion, and forgiveness; these are not inherently linear undertakings. As many who attend therapy have encountered some form of trauma, it is essential to work from a trauma-informed position. Each element of IHT requires the therapist to purposely hold space for the word *trauma* and how it manifests in multitudinous ways. Our clients may not remember an event, but their nervous system will. This may result from an accumulation of events that were never properly processed.

The discomfort felt by clients in session is often a result of unresolved trauma and parts of their life that entail renarrating by means of discussing their metaphorical (and sometimes physical) wounds. Part of the healing process involves relaying experiences or events to the therapist or participating in repetitive storytelling while being and feeling witnessed by the therapist. This differs from classical exposure insofar as rather than sharing trauma repeatedly, clients are disclosing until they feel seen and heard by someone. Clients might be convincing themselves of what has happened in their life, and believing themselves may be part of their healing. Clients learn to process these emotions, accept them, and evolve as people; they both heal within and break cycles.

In early stages of long-term therapy, sessions commence with rapport building, information gathering, and treatment planning. Later sessions offer approaches/techniques and psychoeducation to equip clients for healing. Clients are best supported by theoretical approaches that resonate with their own philosophical leanings; harm can be done if the therapist imposes interventions that do not align with the client's proclivities. Clients may also need to be helped to understand that their issue may "never go away," but the intensity may consequentially lessen. By empowering themselves and their clients to grow in their way of being, therapists empathize rather than internalize their clients' sentiments during session. All learning is mutual and critical to strengthen of the therapeutic alliance. There are five sections of IHT, as shown in Figure 8.1:

1. Exploring Intersectionality
2. Recognizing Encounters with Systemic Oppression
3. Processing Unresolved Trauma
4. Relinquishing Suffering
5. Applying Eastern Healing Practices

The first two sections, *Exploring Intersectionality* and *Recognizing Encounters with Systemic Oppression* require that the therapist and client comprehend the relationship between the individual parts of the client's identity within their overall intersectionality. Unique experiences and hardships are examined through the overlap of these social identities. Chapters 4 to 6 contain constructs relevant to doing so, such as the systemic oppression pyramid (see Figure 4.1). In these two phases of IHT, clients acquire psychoeducation about oppressive systems that have affected their intersectionality. The intersectionality of oppression as defined by Kimberlé Crenshaw (2022) is a means of exploring the dynamics between social identities (i.e., race, class, gender, etc.) and connected systems of oppression (i.e., racism, white supremacy, capitalism, etc.). Oppression is a key factor that allows abuse and assault to occur using social paradigms of power and control, causing many BIPOC to experience multiple forms of trauma throughout their lifetime.

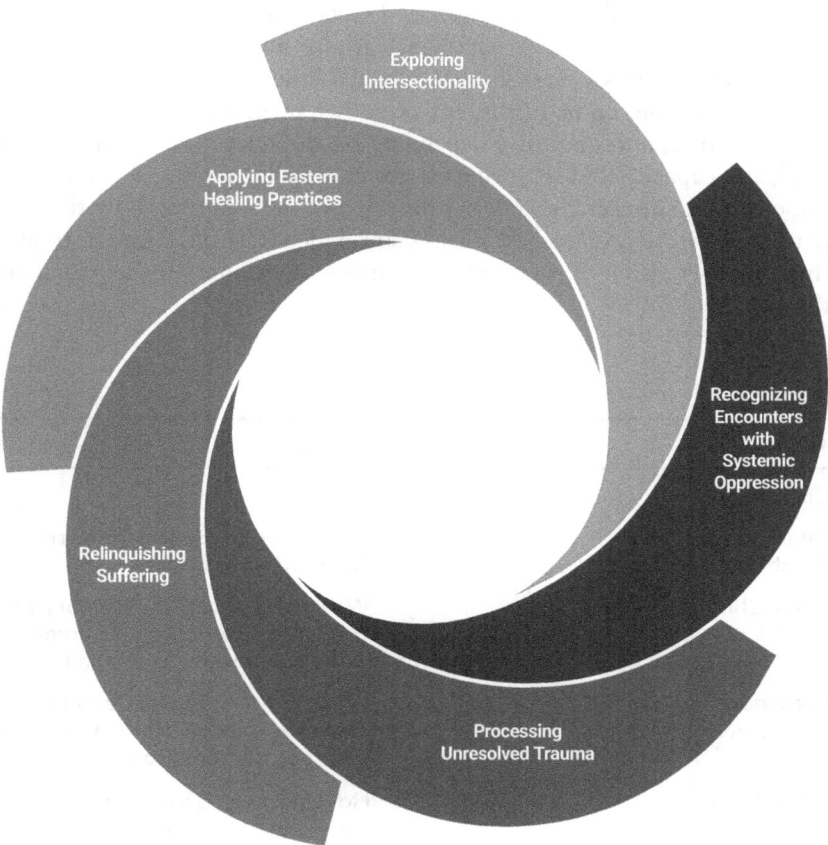

Figure 8.1 Inclusion and healing therapy framework

Drawing from the information in Chapter 4, clients are requested to list aspects of their intersectionality. Clients are also invited to share, deconstruct, and reclaim their cultural narrative and deliberate upon various intersections of their social identities in relation to their experiences and perceptions with systemic inequalities. Information about the client's history is also gathered at this time to understand what emotions may need to be externalized and how the client's story can be renarrated. Clients are asked how silencing their intersectionality contributes to diverse forms of systemic oppression (e.g., racism, capitalism, colonialism, etc.), or how their intersectionality can improve the current sociopolitical landscape and decentre systemic oppression. This conversation is meant to encourage clients to feel safe within each social identity. By understanding a client's intersectionality during therapy, culturally responsive, inclusive, and social justice interventions can be integrated into the therapeutic treatment plan.

Foregrounding Erikson's *Stages of Psychosocial Developmental Model* (1950, 1968), this exercise involves learning about the client's cultural/ ethnic/racial identity across three stages: childhood, adolescence, and adulthood. Each stage can be further broken down (e.g., young adulthood, middle adulthood, and maturity) depending on the relevancy, client's comfort level, and capacity to disclose details about these life phases. Within each of these phases, the therapist takes a deeper dive into learning how these systems of oppression shaped the client's social identities and continue to affect their mindset. Table 8.1 provides examples of prompts to help structure this conversation.

Table 8.1 Life phases and social identity stages

Age	Prompts
Childhood	
Infancy (birth to 18 months)	What is your country of birth? Generational status?
Early Childhood (2 to 3 years)	What is your earliest memory of cultural preservation? At home? Within the ethnic community?
Preschool (3 to 5 years)	What is your recollection of the cultural/ethnic/racial breakdown of your peer/school group?
School Age (6 to 11 years)	How did your family interact with their respective community and host country?
Youth	
Adolescence (12 to 18 years)	Did you experience any form of racism or othering during your teen years?
Adulthood	
Young Adulthood (19 to 40 years)	How were you treated at school or in the workplace?
Middle Adulthood (40 to 65 years)	How did your perceptions of the host country impact cultural preservation in your home environment? What forms of systemic oppression were encountered?
Maturity (65 to death)	What are your reflections regarding your lived experience as an immigrant or BIPOC?

Based on the responses generated from these prompts, this section of IHT concludes with a comprehensive understanding of how clients can shed or externalize core beliefs, which are defined as "fundamental, absolute, and lasting comprehensions that a person develops about him or herself, others, and the world, are constructed from the effort of extracting meaning from significant childhood or formative experiences" (Beck, 2005, 2011; Osmo et al., 2018, p. 67). Examples of core beliefs themes include feelings of inadequacy, lack of belonging, unworthiness, guilt/shame, helplessness, or lack of control.

The third section of IHT, *Processing Unresolved Trauma*, focusses on the relationship between systemic oppression and trauma. Clients are asked to describe how these systems impacted their ancestors as well as their own generation. Trauma can result in the disconnection from oneself, whereas healing is the progression towards reconnecting to oneself. Using Table 2.1, clients identify and discuss relevant forms of experiential trauma. Decolonized strategies such as psychoeducation on culturally relevant trauma responses, understanding links to past ancestral trauma (i.e., colonization, white supremacy, etc.), and psychoeducation on BIPOC mental health oppression support the client's ability to comprehend what is further embedded in their nervous system and how to manage these somatic responses (see Chapter 3 for pertinent exercises). Trauma responding often occurs to protect one's vulnerability, and such vulnerability is necessary to help individuals grieve and heal from past events. This section of IHT supports clients to shift from trauma responding to effective grieving to healing. This can occur by means of locating restorative activities to become resilient, or reframing trauma responses to partake in restorative care.

In the fourth section of the IHT framework, *Relinquishing Suffering*, grief work helps clients to resolve trauma-related anger and shame. Utilizing continuing bonds theory (Klass et al., 1996; Klass, 2006; Lee et al., 2017), clients are supported through a non-linear form of grief work. Continuing bonds are defined by Stroebe and Schut (2005) as "the presence of an ongoing inner relationship with the deceased person by the bereaved individual" (p. 477). Clients are encouraged to forge a continued and renewed bond with their loved one after their passing, moving from mourning the loss to commemorating a new connection (Root & Exline, 2014). This may be comprised of having dreams about the loved one; honouring their loved one's memory; experiencing a sense of presence of the loved one; engaging in conversations with the loved one; sharing narratives about the loved one; and cherishing items that once belonged to the loved one (Field et al., 2013). Alternately or additionally, it may look like disconnecting from their cultural/ethnic/racial community or questioning their cultural identity. Culturally, healing could involve developing a stronger ethnic/racial presence by embodying cultural and religious traditions, understanding ancestral lineage, and relearning a heritage language. This assists with clients feeling connected and making sense of and overcoming loneliness.

Cultural bereavement is a type of grieving that encapsulates a response to the loss of leaving one's country of origin, social structures, cultural values and beliefs, social networks, and self-identity (Bhugra & Becker, 2005). It can include not having a connection to one's culture or the inability to experience it. Examples of different forms of cultural bereavement are colonization and other types of systemic oppression, loss of power and control, collectively grieving historical or racial trauma events, lack of connection to ancestral wisdom, identity confusion, the immigration process, and feeling disconnected to cultural values and traditions (Yoon et al., 2022). Using components of the cultural bereavement interview (Eisenbruch, 1990), clients are asked to explore the following personal and collective losses:

1. Guilt
2. Dreams
3. Ghosts or spirits from the past
4. Past routines in the homeland
5. Continuing experiences of family and past
6. The comfort derived from religious beliefs
7. Personal experiences of death and funerals
8. The comfort obtained from participation in religious gatherings
9. Anxieties, morbid thoughts, and anger in response to separation from the homeland
10. Memories of a family in the homeland and clarity with which appearance of relations is recalled

In IHT, grief is also examined through the lens of Buddhist psychology, especially when differentiating the disparities or similarities between ancestral and host cultural practices. I apply teachings from Buddhist psychology, such as the Four Noble Truths, the Middle Path, clinging, and forgiveness to help clients understand the distinction between trauma, grief, and suffering (Neimeyer & Young-Eisendrath, 2015; Sodhi, 2017). For example, grief work is introduced, as are strategies to reconcile anger, shame, and guilt. Clients explore situational grief, name feelings/emotions, and contemplate the interplay within their current life. Lastly, information about forgiveness and self-compassion are examined (Kornfield, 2008; Neff, 2015; Sodhi, 2021).

The fifth and final section of IHT, *Applying Eastern Healing Practices* (e.g., continuity of community care, inner work, etc.), identifies how healing is transmitted, healing practices, and perceptions of healers within the community and society (Egnew, 2005). Healing, as described by Maté and Maté (2022), involves moving towards a place of wholeness and can be considered a lifelong trajectory. As intersectional beings, some of one's social identities may achieve healing with more or less support than others. Additionally, healing includes navigating the zone of proximal development (ZPD), an "interpersonal space where minds meet and new understandings can arise through collaborative interaction and inquiry" (Cummins, 1996, p. 26). Healing is an opportunity for individuals to move in their ZPDs and create new meaning about their healing while instantaneously grieving dimensions of personal loss and trauma (Sodhi, 2017; Vygotsky, 1978).

Maté and Maté (2022) share the 4 A's (healing principles): authenticity, agency, acceptance, and anger (healthy). What truly resonates for my BIPOC clients is the importance of taking initiative and control in one's healing process reflected by the second A (agency). Maté and Maté (2022) express that it is those who take matters into their own hands and confront adversity in their life who will have more success at healing from their trauma. Agency aligns with the notions of being a cycle breaker and taking risks to avoid perpetuating intergenerational cycles. To break cycles, however, individuals must be confident in their way of being and willing to assert and set boundaries to protect themselves from those who might sabotage or create an unnecessary detour in their healing process.

Akin to grief, healing can be non-linear or cyclical. For example, I present the "Trauma-Healing Continuum" (See Figure 3.3) to clients for them to comprehend that clinical work will require them to process their traumatic event, identify stages of grief, employ grounding and reframing techniques, recognize personal growth, move towards acceptance, and appreciate that healing is ongoing. We also recount what our ancestors have taught us to support long-term healing; communal healing is inherent to BIPOC trauma work. "When we meet our needs within the community, we must compromise less with harmful systems. Community care helps insulate us from white supremist capitalism that wants to tear us apart" (Oluo, 2021). Clients learn how systematic/structural oppression dehumanizes people and hinders access to mental health supports; they also learn to feel seen and prepared to participate in a decolonized community mental healthcare model while recognizing and externalizing oppression. Clients tap into the power of their elders and ancestors, locating spiritual wholeness resulting from the suffering and reconciliation of groups. Community supports specific for BIPOC, therapeutic approaches (established in Eastern ideologies), and personalized treatment plans for BIPOC generate and encourage empowerment and accountability for long-term growth, healing, and connection.

Chapter 9 applies inclusion and healing therapy to the narratives shared in Part 3 to illustrate the versatility of IHT.

References

Beck, J. S. (2005). *Cognitive therapy for challenging problems: What to do when the basics don't work*. Guilford Press.

Beck, J. S. (2011). *Cognitive behavior therapy: Basics and beyond* (2nd ed.). Guilford Press.

Bhugra, D., & Becker, M. (2005). Migration, cultural bereavement and cultural identity. *World Psychiatry: Official Journal of the World Psychiatric Association, 4*(1), 18–24.

Crenshaw, K. (2022). *Intersectionality: Essential writings*. The New Press.

Cummins, J. (1996). *Negotiating identities: Education for empowerment in a diverse society*. California Association of Bilingual Education.

Dossey, B. M., & Keegan, L. (2009). *Holistic nursing: A handbook for practice* (5th ed.). Jones & Bartlett.

Egnew, T. R. (2005). The meaning of healing: Transcending suffering. *Annals of Family Medicine, 3*(3), 255–262.

Eisenbruch, M. (1990). The cultural bereavement interview: A new clinical research approach for refugees. *The Psychiatric Clinics of North America, 13*(4), 715–735.

Erikson, E. H. (1950). *Childhood and society*. W.W. Norton.

Erikson, E. H. (1968). *Identity: Youth and crisis*. W.W. Norton.

Field, N. P., Packman, W., Ronen, R., Pries, A., Davies, B., & Kramer, R. (2013). Types of continuing bonds expression and its comforting versus distressing nature: Implications for adjustment among bereaved mothers. *Death Studies, 37*, 889–912.

Harris, R. (2008). *The happiness trap: How to stop struggling and start living: A guide to ACT*. Trumpeters Publishers.

Klass, D. (2006). Continuing conversation about continuing bonds. *Death Studies, 30*(9), 843–858.

Klass, D., Silverman, P. R., & Nickman, S. L. (Eds.). (1996). *Continuing bonds: New understandings of grief*. Taylor & Francis.

Kornfield, J. (2008). *The art of forgiveness, lovingkindness, and peace*. W.W. Norton.

Kottler, J. A. (2022). *On being a therapist* (6th ed.). Oxford University Press.

Lee, W.-L., Hou, Y.-C., & Lin, Y.-S. (2017). Revisiting the continuing bonds theory: The cultural uniqueness of the Bei Dao phenomenon in Taiwanese widows/widowers. *Qualitative Health Research, 27*(12), 1892–1904.

Maté, G., & Maté, D. (2022). *The myth of normal: Trauma, illness, and healing in a toxic culture*. Knopf Canada.

Motiño, A., Saiz, J., Sánchez-Iglesias, I., Salazar, M., Barsotti, T. J., Goldsby, T. L., Chopra, D., & Mills, P. J. (2021). Cross-Cultural analysis of spiritual bypass: A comparison between Spain and Honduras. *Frontiers in Psychology, 12*, 658739.

Naeem, F., Tuck, A., Mutta, B. Dillon, P., Thandi, G., Kassam, A., Farah, N., Ashraf, A. A., Husain, M. I., Husain, M. O., Vasiliadis, H.-M., Sanches, M., Munshi, T., Abbott, M., Watters, N., Kidd, S. A., Ayub, M., & McKenzie, K. (2021). Protocol for a multi-phase, mixed methods study to develop and evaluate culturally adapted CBT to improve community mental health services for Canadians of South Asian origin. *Trials, 22*, 600.

Neff, K. (2015). *Self-compassion: The proven power of being kind to yourself*. William Morrow and Company.

Neimeyer, R. A., & Young-Eisendrath, P. (2015). Assessing a Buddhist treatment for bereavement and loss: The mustard seed project. *Death Studies*, *39*(5), 263–273.

Oluo, I. (2021). *Is it self-care or is it capitalism?* Retrieved November 5, 2021, from https://ijeomaoluo.substack.com/p/is-it-self-care-or-is-it-capitalism

O'Mara, J., & Richter, A. (2017). *Global diversity & inclusion benchmarks: Standards for organisations around the world.* Retrieved August 4, 2022, from https://centreforglobalinclusion.org/wp-content/uploads/2017/09/GDIB-V.090517.pdf

Osmo, F., Duran, V., Wenzel, A., de Oliveira, I. R., Nepomuceno, S., Madeira, M., & Menezes, I. (2018). The negative core beliefs inventory: Development and psychometric properties. *Journal of Cognitive Psychotherapy*, *32*(1), 67–84.

Root, B. L., & Exline, J. J. (2014). The role of continuing bonds in coping with grief: Overview and future directions. *Death Studies*, *38*(1–5), 1–8.

Seeley, K. M. (2004). Short-term intercultural psychotherapy: Ethnographic inquiry. *Social Work*, *49*(1), 121–130.

Sodhi, P. K. (2017). *Exploring immigrant and sexual minority mental health: Reconsidering multiculturalism.* Routledge.

Sodhi, P. K. (2021). The Sikh spirit of Chardi Kala (resilience) as a cure for grief. Panelist. *Parliament of the World's Religions virtual conference*, October 16–18, 2021.

Stroebe, M., & Schut, H. (2005). To continued or relinquish bonds: A review of consequences for the bereaved. *Death Studies*, *29*(6), 477–494.

Trungpa, C. (2010). *The sanity we are born with: A Buddhist approach to psychology.* Shambala.

Vygotsky, L. S. (1978). *Mind in society: The development of higher psychological processes.* Harvard University Press.

Yoon, M. S., Zhang, N., & Feyissa, I. F. (2022). Cultural Bereavement and mental distress: Examination of the cultural bereavement framework through the case of Ethiopian refugees living in South Korea. *Healthcare*, *10*(2), 201.

Chapter 9

Revisiting BIPOC Narratives

The final chapter of this part of the book applies inclusion and healing therapy (IHT) to the narratives from Part 3. Case conceptualization summaries, treatment plans, and exercises explicate how to effectively provide decolonized trauma-informed techniques to BIPOC.

John and Segal (2015) wrote:

Case conceptualization (also called case formulation) refers to the clinician's collective understanding of the client's presenting problems as viewed through a particular theoretical orientation; as defined by the biological, psychological, and social contexts of the client; and as supported by a body of research and practice that links a set of co-occurring symptoms to a diagnosis and, ultimately, a treatment plan.

(p. 1)

Notably, a viable case conceptualization is supported by diverse theoretical orientations (e.g., psychoanalytic theory, narrative therapy, cognitive behavioural therapy) or can be problem or condition-based to amalgamate aspects of the client's narrative into a cohesive format (Kilcullen & Day, 2018). What is frequently missing from case conceptualization are the cultural and biopsychosocial variables linked to one's intersectionality; these variables are integral to a decolonized analysis process.

During my therapy sessions, I purposefully decolonize and simplify the initial meeting to minimize paperwork and maximize supportive dialogue. The client's history is heard and collected at the beginning of the therapeutic process by means of objective, positive, and culturally responsive/affirming history taking. Rather than setting Western capitalist goals with my BIPOC clients, we create therapeutic aspirations. To ensure intersectional components are unpacked, I apply prompts from Table 9.1 to generate pertinent discourse about the client's narrative and reason(s) for seeking therapy.

DOI: 10.4324/9781003216568-14

Table 9.1 Initial meeting criteria

Initial Meeting Criteria	Topics
Cultural definition of the presenting problem(s)	What brings the client to therapy? Discuss: origins of the problem, precursors, strengths, barriers, and risk factors.
Gather history and background information	Additional information that may need to be elaborated upon.
Risk screening	Toward self (suicidality concerns: thoughts, ideations, plans, actions) or others.
Cultural and psychosocial variables	Relationship status; migratory experiences; family dynamics (family of origin experiences); educational/training background; employment history; community membership; host culture perceptions; social supports; previous counselling/therapy; history of trauma/abuse; addictions or mental health issues; lifestyle: nutrition, sleep hygiene, and exercise; and hobbies/self-care protocols.
Therapeutic aspirations	Collaborate with client; what are their intentions for therapy?
Recommendations and treatment plan	Next steps: strategies to achieve therapeutic aspirations with the use of relevant therapeutic techniques/approaches and psychoeducation.

Again, the initial meeting is not highly structured and instead can be viewed as a collective venture. By including humanistic doctrines like Rogers' necessary conditions for therapy (Rogers, 1961, 1989), the primary focus is strengthening the alliance rather than the actual therapeutic process (Paré, 2013).

The works of Kilcullen and Day (2018) and Sperry and Sperry (2012, 2020) inform this chapter, as both of their formats validate attributes that support a biopsychosocial, culturally responsive, and decolonized case conceptualization process. Kilcullen and Day (2018) suggest including analysis of self, family and kinship connectedness, social connectedness, and cultural connectedness, which also summarize individual, community, social, historical, and political aspects. Further, content from Sperry and Sperry (2020) is highlighted, particularly predispositions such as biological history (i.e., family history of mental or physical health issues), psychological content (i.e., concerns of maintaining friendship, assertiveness issues), social connectedness (i.e., childhood issues, financial concerns, parenting style disparities), and cultural connectedness (i.e., acculturation matters, adapting to a new country).

Table 9.2 BIPOC case conceptualization summaries

BIPOC	Self	Family and Kinship Connectedness	Biological History	Psychological Context	Social Connectedness	Cultural Connectedness
Jamal (he/him)	Unpack generational trauma and racism. Overcome racial guilt and shame. Coping strategies: soccer, piano, and productive allyship with Black Lives Matter.	Appreciate the pressure of being the familial cycle breaker and carrying the burden of previous ancestors.	Learn more about how the impact racial trauma and police brutality had on his family and now himself.	Relearn trust and safety as a black male. Anticipatory anxiety and fear of how he will be treated.	Access support from his family in comprehending their coping strategies. Educating future generations about the triumphs and hardships of being a young black male.	Refamiliarize himself with Nigerian culture, spiritual beliefs, and healing practices. Become a member of the black association at his university.
Mikom (they/them)	Revisit the impacts of forced assimilation, cultural genocide, and colonialism on Mikom's intersectionality. Coping strategies: painting; alcohol and drug use.	Reconcile the loss of their father and the embedded years of intergenerational trauma in their family.	Explore the affect of colonialism on their extended family, understand their grandmother's panic attacks and psychosis, as well as their mother's bouts of depression.	Confront embracing the two-spirit identification and making sense of their traumatic past.	Seek different forms of guidance from the members of the reserve and the 2SLGBTQQIA+ community in Halifax, Nova Scotia, and other local resources to overcome their substance use disorder.	Reconnect with family members, including their sisters, mother, and grandmother. Give back to the reserve they resided upon; continue to learn from members of the reserve.

Prem (he/him)	Questions whether living in Canada is worthwhile; experience with systemic oppression and barriers and grieve multiple losses. Coping strategies: work, community involvement, and investing time in his children.	Learn to forgive the past, particularly his father's treatment towards him and having no regrets about moving to Canada.	Come to terms with his father's methods of discipline, mother's passing, and not being able to support from afar during assorted familial hardships.	Ambivalent about moving abroad, given the diverse barriers he experienced during his lifetime. Accept his bicultural identity and ability to deflect everyday racism.	Spend time with his wife, family, and close friends. Discuss his narrative of survival with his grandchildren, who will continue to learn from his immigrant legacy.	Recognize that moving to Canada was the best decision that he could have made at that time. Connect with community, where nostalgia, co-regulating, and collective grief can transpire.
Isla (she/her)	Locate a culturally responsive psychotherapist to help with C-PTSD. Coping strategies: grounding and visions of having her own business so that she can provide for her children.	Respect her parents' intentions in the past, try to forgive them for their guidance, and overcome abandonment wounds.	Acknowledge that she carries vicarious trauma from her uncle's death and grief from the passing of her stillborn child and challenging marriage.	Create silos for the countless tragic events that happened throughout her lifetime. Try to reframe and move forward from these traumas.	Rebuild relationship with parents and siblings; learn to trust again. Overcome parentification from the past and prevent repeating these patterns with her children.	Accept that she lives in a country where there is perpetual fear and concerns around safety. Actualize the limitations of living within this cultural space.

(Continued)

Table 9.2 (Continued)

BIPOC	Self	Family and Kinship Connectedness	Biological History	Psychological Context	Social Connectedness	Cultural Connectedness
Yin (she/her)	Confront the historical and cultural trauma specific to her Asian heritage; unlearn model minority myth. Coping strategies: playing the flute and drawing.	Admire her parents for migrating from China to provide a better life for her family and being able to move to the United States where her aunt lives. Help her family rebuild their life after experiencing trauma in China.	Compartmentalize her family's trauma and z. Process years of trauma so that she can actualize her potential.	Assert herself, but still feels silenced. Only taken seriously due to her ethnicity and strong work ethic.	Devote time with her parents, brother, grandparents, and extended family. Take the opportunity to reframe individuals' perceptions about Chinese culture and immigrants.	Develop a positive association with her ethnicity. Acquire self-compassion for how she was treated throughout her lifetime for being Asian.

IHT Treatment Plans

Two comprehensive tables are provided; the first table captures case conceptualization summaries, and the other table discusses strategies relevant to the IHT framework.

Table 9.2 illustrates case conceptualization summaries of the BIPOC clients from Part 3; it may help to reread these vignettes prior to continuing this chapter to refresh your memory. The table is comprised of six categories: self, family and kinship connectedness, biological history, psychological context, social connectedness, and cultural connectedness.

Complementing information from Table 9.2, Table 9.3 offers insight and strategies applicable to the inclusion and healing therapy framework (e.g., exploring intersectionality, recognizing encounters with systemic oppression, processing unresolved trauma, relinquishing suffering, and Eastern healing practices). Each BIPOC client would receive a comprehensive initial meeting; this affords time for the therapist to review confidentiality protocols in addition to the content noted in Table 9.3. A detailed description of inclusion and healing therapy treatment plans follows with select referencing to Table 9.2.

Jamal

Jamal's purpose for seeking therapy is twofold:

1. Overcome years of intergenerational trauma stored in his nervous system.
2. Receive culturally affirming therapy to further understand and process the police brutality he experienced.

Jamal's sessions commenced with an in-depth exploration of his intersectionality and his associated perceptions. I provided him with psychoeducation and definitions of intersectionality. I then asked him to disclose his most pronounced social identities; he identifies as a 21-year-old black bicultural second-generation Nigerian immigrant, descendant of slaves, Ivy League university student, athlete, and heterosexual cisgender male. Jamal was able to share his perception of each identity and remarked that words such as privilege, oppression, determination, and resiliency overlap within his intersecting identities.

He recognized the power and privilege garnered to him through being a heterosexual male attending an esteemed university; however, combined with these attributes, his race and slave ancestry both shackle him with stereotypes, barriers, and forms of systemic oppression, such as white supremacy, colonialism, capitalism, racism, and discrimination. He was hoping to

Table 9.3 Application of inclusion and healing therapy framework

BIPOC Client	Exploring Intersectionality	Recognizing Encounters with Systemic Oppression	Processing Unresolved Trauma	Relinquishing Suffering	Applying Eastern Healing Practices
Jamal (he/him)	Identifies as a 21-year-old, black bicultural second-generation Nigerian immigrant, descendant of slaves, Ivy League university student, athlete, and heterosexual cisgender male.	White supremacy, colonialism, capitalism, racism, and discrimination.	C-PTSD, systemic trauma, racial trauma, and intergenerational trauma. **Strategies:** – Autonomic nervous system ladder – Individual/family trauma framework	***Continuing bonds theory:*** Reconnecting with Nigerian heritage and black community on campus. ***Cultural bereavement:*** Reclamation of past traumas (enslavement) and current treatment as a black male living in America. ***Buddhist psychology:*** Finding the Middle Path towards acceptance.	Map trauma-healing continuum and constructs pertaining to the stages of forgiveness.
Mikom (they/them)	Identifies as a 32-year-old two-spirit Mi'kmaq individual, member of the K'jipuktuk (Halifax) 2SLGBTQQIA+ community, descendant of residential school survivors, and youngest child.	Colonialism, white supremacy, racial inequity, racism, and discrimination.	Colonial trauma, developmental trauma, intersectional trauma, and intergenerational trauma. **Strategies:** – Inner BIPOC child wounds – Cultural "never good enough" cycle	***Continuing bonds theory:*** Grieving the loss of their father at a young age. ***Cultural bereavement:*** Understand the root of their trauma, specifically in relation to the residential school system; explore identity confusion. ***Buddhist psychology:*** Silo grief, attachment, and suffering.	Complete the resiliency model and reclaim their cultural narrative.

| **Prem (he/him)** | Identifies as a 90-year-old first-generation South Asian immigrant, 1947 Partition of India/Pakistan survivor, father of three children, retired educator, and heterosexual cisgender male. | Colonialism in India and Canada, racial inequity, racism, and discrimination. | Colonial trauma, cultural trauma, developmental trauma, migratory trauma, systemic trauma, racial trauma, collective trauma, intergenerational trauma. **Strategies:** – Culturally relevant trauma responses – Situational grief | ***Continuing bonds theory:*** Commemorate late family members and the influence they had on his life. ***Cultural bereavement:*** Come to terms with the sacrifices made to immigrate to a country, the lack of relationship with his father, experience systemic oppression, and feelings of disconnect from ancestral culture. ***Buddhist psychology:*** Extricate and reframe clinging mindset and grieve the guilt experienced due to immigrating. | Discuss silencing the inner cultural critic and intersectional healing. |

(Continued)

Table 9.3 (Continued)

BIPOC Client	Exploring Intersectionality	Recognizing Encounters with Systemic Oppression	Processing Unresolved Trauma	Relinquishing Suffering	Applying Eastern Healing Practices
Isla (she/her)	Identifies as a 40-year-old Latine, lower class, separated mother of three children, and heterosexual cisgender female.	Patriarchy and capitalism.	Developmental trauma, C-PTSD, and systemic trauma. **Strategies:** – Codependent-interdependent spectrum – Negotiating boundaries within a cultural space	***Continuing bonds theory:*** Grieve the loss of her stillborn child. ***Cultural bereavement:*** Reconnect with familial values and culture that was forsaken at the time of her marriage. Contend with loss and control in her life. ***Buddhist psychology:*** Learn to forgive herself and others for her life choices.	Identify grounding techniques, glimmers, and self-soothing exercises; examine the trauma-healing continuum.
Yin (she/her)	Identifies as a 34-year-old second-generation Chinese immigrant, professor at an American university, and heterosexual cisgender female.	Racial inequity, racism, discrimination, and hate crimes.	Cultural trauma, developmental trauma, migratory trauma, systemic trauma, racial trauma, collective trauma, and intergenerational trauma. **Strategies:** – Culturally relevant trauma responses – Ethnic guilt	***Continuing bonds theory:*** Make peace with Chinese culture and the stigma associated with being Asian. ***Cultural bereavement:*** Address her post-migration challenges, experiences with racism, and hate crimes. ***Buddhist psychology:*** Revisit the Four Noble Truths to comprehend and renounce suffering from her life.	Create a cultural safety road map and explore intersectional healing.

have a fresh start or *tabula rasa* (clean slate) upon enrolling in university, but these oppressive systems seemed to have followed him as he carries ancestral pain and hurt from the past.

Using a prompt from "Life Phases and Social Identity Stages" in Table 8.1, Jamal was asked: "How did your family interact with their respective community and host country?" Jamal was able to confirm that his family kept to themselves within the host country, but also connected with other Nigerian immigrants for annual holidays and on the weekends. As part of his beliefs around breaking intergenerational cycles, he chose not to meet as often with Nigerian community peers and instead invested more time and energy with his mostly white varsity soccer team. In retrospect, Jamal confessed that he may have internalized racism to fit in more so that he could feel more accepted by members of the host culture. He believed that if he succeeded in soccer, Ivy League universities would look past his race and oppressive past and view him as a talented student and athlete.

Jamal may have subscribed to covering (Goffman, 1963); that is, he concealed a part of his identity. He may have even succumbed to code-switching where one leads a dual identity to blend into the host culture (Sodhi, 2017). Both these coping strategies can be exhausting and may require proving oneself both at home and in the host culture to make the host country more hospitable. Jamal reconsidered showing up authentically for himself; he decided it was important to believe in himself, speak with confidence, and have faith in his abilities. This led to pinpointing embedded core beliefs. Jamal was asked what core beliefs are relevant to systemic oppression that he would like to deconstruct; Jamal identified guilt/shame for not being more involved and connected to his Nigerian community and unworthiness within the host country. He now believes both core beliefs distorted his self-perception and his familial interactions. By externalizing these core beliefs, Jamal would like to replace these with educating future generations about the lived experience of being a young black male, reconnecting with family, Nigerian culture, spiritual beliefs, healing practices, and possibly becoming a member of the black association at his university.

Having a better understanding of how systemic oppression impacted his intersectionality, Jamal was ready to confront his personal and ancestral traumas. When presented with Table 2.1, "Types of Trauma," Jamal named complex post-traumatic stress disorder (C-PTSD), systemic trauma, racial trauma, and intergenerational trauma. He recognized that his family has a significant history with trauma, particularly being enslaved and oppressed for several centuries. We proceeded to map Jamal's autonomic nervous system states and associated emotions using a polyvagal framework (Dana, 2021; Porges, 2011). After reviewing the three states on the "Autonomic Nervous System Ladder" (See Figure 3.1),

Jamal immediately gravitated towards the dorsal vagal state where he claimed he was shutting down, feeling disconnected from himself and the world, and immobilized. I explained to him that "shifting states" to reach the ventral vagal state is possible and would require Jamal to internally access some "sympathetic mobilized energy" (Dana, 2018) to expand his window of tolerance. To prevent dysregulation he could implement somatic work such as breathing techniques, exercising, and body scans to cultivate awareness of the hurt stored in his body.

Upon establishing stabilization and affect regulation, Jamal felt more inner calm and connection. He was presented with the "Individual/Family Trauma Framework" shown in Figure 3.4 and was asked to separate his traumas from his family's trauma. As provided in Chapter 3, individual and family trauma intersects within a collectivist context. His responses are written within Figure 9.1:

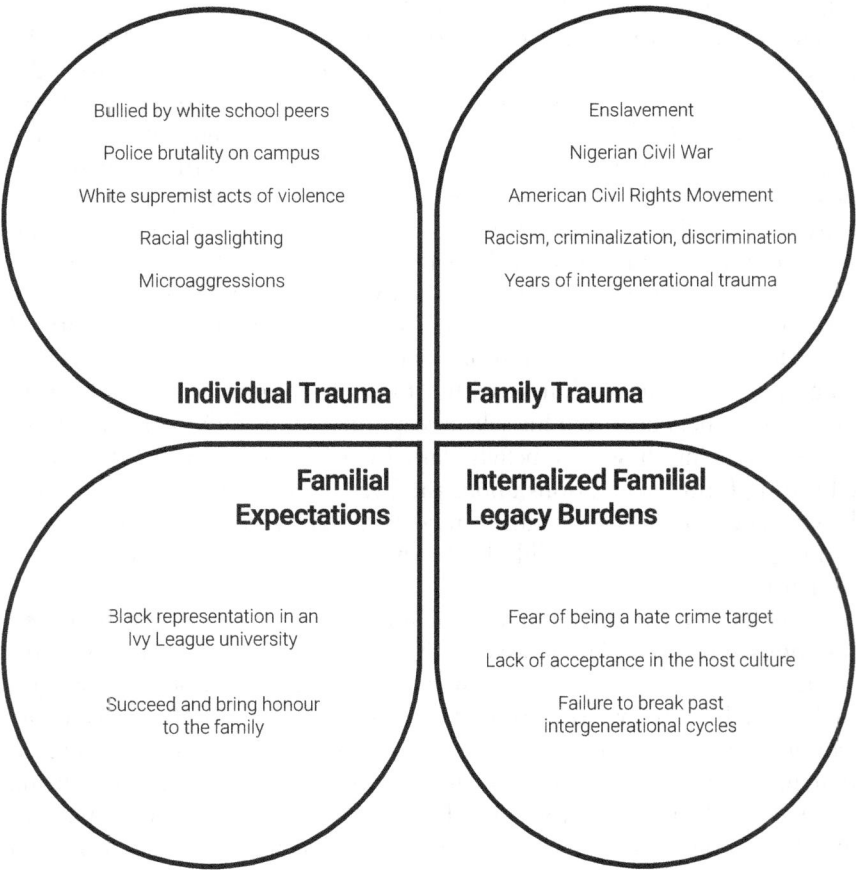

Figure 9.1 Jamal's individual/family trauma framework

Jamal acknowledges the link between his personal and family's traumas and how these events have shaped his intersectionality. His family has been marginalized for centuries, leaving them feeling excluded in the host culture. They have been subjected to abuse over the years, wanting to make a name for themselves. Jamal desperately attempted to break these cycles by trying to fit in with the white culture, being the first in his family to attend university, and hoping to make his family proud. He experienced vicarious trauma because of his father's mistreatment in the workplace, his brother's incarceration, and was also traumatized by minimization of his bullying by white school peers. He never wanted to be a victim of hate crime.

Jamal was able to let go of the internalized familial legacy burdens. This was not his responsibility anymore. For several years, he held onto the ancestral shame and guilt and believed he was meant to change his family history and destiny. His trauma was indeed distinct from his family's trauma and transpired under different contexts; it shaped his intersectionality, specifically the layers of oppression and his slave ancestry, all of which taught him to be humble and grateful, but also not good enough or accepted within a primarily white society. Jamal's motive was to reauthor his family's narrative so that these past social identities could be viewed as events that have brought intergenerational resiliency to the family rather than oppression.

To continue relinquishing suffering, Jamal acknowledged his need to reconnect with his Nigerian heritage and the black community on campus, as well as his need to reclaim and reframe the past traumas (enslavement), stereotypes, and discrimination that impact him as a black male. He was able to do so by locating the Middle Path towards acceptance (Monteiro et al., 2017), a balance between the reasonable mind and emotional mind, when these feelings of inadequacy surface. This exercise empowered Jamal the resiliency that he has inherited and his ability to look beyond the racial ignorance and colonization that exists in our society.

For the final section of the IHT framework, Eastern healing practices, Jamal reinforced his progress with a reflection informed by the "Trauma-Healing Continuum" (See Figure 3.3) to process a traumatic event, identify stages of grief, participate in grounding and reframing exercises, recognize personal growth, move towards acceptance, and believe that healing is ongoing. Jamal applied Figure 3.3 to the police brutality event, identified with the stage of shock, integrated grounding techniques that resonate with him (e.g., exercising, body scans), reframe and remind himself that this event is separate from his family's trauma, and observing that he has made progress in not internalizing this event as an attack on his lineage as he gradually tries to shift towards some form of acceptance throughout this continuous healing process.

Jamal punctuated his healing by "letting go by engaging in cognitive reframing and understanding the duality of the situation" and "moving forward and learning from these experiences; actualizing a compassionate way of being," both of which he connected to the "Stages of Forgiveness" in Chapter 3. The purpose of this exercise was for Jamal to forgive and embody self-compassion and loving kindness. Jamal was provided with a personalized treatment plan that offered him ways to access inner strength, empowerment, and ancestral wisdom and to recognize that decolonized healing from trauma is a lifelong process of personal growth and development.

Mikom

Mikom would like to attend therapy:

1. To understand their substance use disorder.
2. To learn about how past abandonment was creating personal obstacles in their life.

To gain a better understanding of Mikom, we discussed their intersectionality and affiliated perceptions. I imparted psychoeducation and definitions of intersectionality. They were then asked to name relevant social identities; they identify as a 32-year-old two-spirit Mi'kmaq member of the *K'jipuktuk* (Halifax) 2SLGBTQQIA+ community, of residential school ancestry, and the youngest child in the family. Mikom disclosed their perception of each identity specifying that oppression, colonization, and discrimination were embedded within their identities. They comprehended that there was a clear interplay between their social identities and the varied systemic oppression which they experienced during their lifetime. Their lineage has been repeatedly silenced by colonialism, white supremacy, racial inequity, racism, and discrimination; these trauma wounds remained active in Mikom's nervous system. They claimed that smoking cannabis helped ground them to the point where they could no longer feel any ancestral pain. Unfortunately, the shame of using alcohol and drugs continued to estrange them from family.

A prompt from Table 8.1, "Life Phases and Social Identity Stages," was used to expand on Mikom's internalized oppression. They were asked, "What is your earliest memory of cultural preservation?" Mikom shared their earliest cultural memory, which included both of their parents at a drum circle. They recalled sitting on their father's shoulders at the age of four as he translated and described the symbolism of this ceremony. Their father said that one day they would be able to participate in the drum circle to connect and communicate with ancestors and the spiritual world. This event was the start of Mikom's captivation of the Mi'kmaq culture and their desire to learn from members of the reserve. Smudging was of particular interest to Mikom, and while living on the reserve, they practiced smudging to cleanse themselves and their space of negative energy. Once Mikom moved to Halifax, they chose not to continue this practice of smudging so as to assimilate to the colonial ways.

After recounting this childhood memory and false promise made by their father, Mikom's sense of rejection from their father became pronounced. Similarly, they identified with the following core beliefs: unworthiness for not being wanted by his father and feelings of inadequacy due to their addiction to alcohol and drugs to cope with past traumas and being abandoned. Both core beliefs caused Mikom to question their place within their family and supress their sadness with substances. They wanted to challenge and replace these core beliefs by accessing guidance from trusted members of the reserve, attending culturally and 2SLGBTQ-QIA+ affirming substance use programs in Halifax, reconnecting with their grandmother, mother, and sisters, and eventually spending time and supporting two-spirit adolescents on the reserve.

This awareness has allowed Mikom to reconcile their understanding of how systemic oppression has influenced their intersectionality in addition to feeling somewhat grounded in their next steps towards recovery. Mikom then began processing unresolved trauma. Mikom was asked to review Table 2.1, "Types of Trauma," and indicated which kinds of traumas were experienced. Mikom pointed to colonial trauma, developmental trauma (Adverse Childhood Experiences), intersectional trauma, and intergenerational trauma. What seemed most evident for Mikom were "Inner BIPOC Child Wounds" (introduced in Chapter 3) they had experienced throughout their life. We explored the abandonment, trust, and neglect wounds, supporting Mikom as they processed the hurt and pain of having an estranged father, and validating their emotions surrounding these hardships.

Mikom remarked that their father was very present in their life until they were seven-years-old, at which point their father vanished without saying goodbye. Initially, Mikom's mother said that their father needed to go away to visit a relative in Shelburne on the South Shore of Nova Scotia for a few days. As the weeks passed, Mikom started questioning their mother about their father's whereabouts; each time they were met with a different response. As the one-year mark approached, Mikom demanded again, and finally their mother told the truth, that their father got in a heated argument with a senior member of the reserve because of his excessive drinking and was told to stop these habits or leave the reserve. Mikom's father was unable to cope without substances, so he left the reserve. Due to his feelings of inadequacy and shame, he did not say goodbye to Mikom or his daughters.

For years, Mikom tried to understand why this happened, but in turn, they internalized the messaging of not being good enough to be their father's child. Mikom felt lost without their father. They particularly feared being alone, not being wanted, and did not trust close family members. We worked through these wounds using a decolonized approach (Sodhi, 2021b). We collectively identified that cultural expectations from others intersected with Mikom's core belief of unworthiness. They wondered if they were good enough for their father or even capable of preserving Mi'kmaq traditions, even though they continued to attend Indigenous events on the reserve long after their father left.

Finally, Mikom and I discussed attachment styles and how Mikom previously connected with other family members. Mikom stated that developing a closeness with their mother was challenging due to her dishonesty concerning their father's departure from the reserve. Upon reviewing the four types of attachment styles (i.e., secure, anxious avoidant, and disorganized) (Bowlby, 1988), Mikom disclosed that they have an anxious attachment style due to their fear of abandonment, difficulty trusting others, lack of self-care, need for constant reassurance, and feelings of insecurity within relationships (Heller, 2019). We explored this attachment style through a decolonized lens and whether these attributes contribute to intergenerational trauma and associated grief. Mikom was asked what events were internalized or compartmentalized. Mikom affirmed that the ancestral trauma consisting of forced assimilation, cultural genocide, witnessing family members' mental health issues, and the sudden departure of their father left a substantial impression on them and that decades of suffering resulted.

In the past, Mikom tried to reconcile with these traumas; however, thoughts and emotions associated with these events manifested in tremendous grief, sadness, pain, and inadequacy, particularly with the lack of a father figure in their life. We reviewed the "Cultural Never Good Enough Cycle" (see Figure 3.6) and how the inner critic reminds Mikom of their traumatic past compounded by the absence of a father. These intrusive thoughts affect Mikom's confidence and increase their resentment around the lack of control they have concerning these life events. They become overwhelmed and anxious and start to internalize guilt and shame for harbouring intergenerational trauma and negative feelings towards their father. To cope, Mikom initially would paint; however, this hobby did not alleviate the inner pain that worsened over time. Mikom was introduced to alcohol and cannabis by older peers on the reserve and noticed that they were able to escape these negative feelings and temporarily feel good about themselves. They were aware that substances were not a long-term solution, yet these habits spanned almost two decades, and Mikom desired other coping strategies.

I recommended some personalized coping methods to Mikom. My intention was to help them become resilient by managing and reducing their anxiety and augmenting their self-confidence. Mikom agreed that learning about inner BIPOC child wounds was very helpful in understanding their abandonment wound. They started surrounding themselves with a more supportive network, connecting with family and friends from the reserve, and holding space for self-compassion and patience with learning and healing taking place.

To further enhance Mikom's healing process, we examined the role of suffering in their life. Their affiliation with the reserve shifted when Mikom learned the truth about their father and considered whether this also instigated their sisters leaving the reserve. Since initiating therapy together, Mikom began commemorating the loss of their father by practicing hand drums and learning to paint nature scenes found close to the reserve. One of Mikom's fondest memories of their father was watching him paint Indigenous artwork and display these pieces in the family home. From all the previous therapeutic conversations, Mikom now has a clearer understanding of the multifaceted and complicated origins of their mental health difficulties. They are aware that the intergenerational trauma bequeathed by the residential school system can affect all subsequent generations. Their developmental trauma of losing their father and intersectional trauma of identifying as a two-spirit individual also impacted their current way of being. Mikom has had some success with compartmentalizing grief, which they now know is the root of their suffering and linked to their attachment style (Thich, 1999).

Examining the role of suffering in Mikom's life led to understanding their pain using the "Resiliency Model" (see Figure 3.5). The activating event was the loss of their father and resultant suffering from lacking such parental guidance in life and culture. We discussed how this past suffering was represented in Mikom's current life. Mikom mentioned that their hurt was so deeply ingrained that it was almost unbearable to stay on the same reserve that rejected their father. Mikom was asked whether they have ever participated in collective healing and if this may be a means to overcoming their hurt. Mikom was not opposed to this option, appreciated the value of healing as a community, and believed that there were pre-emptive steps required to undertake such a process. To facilitate collective healing, Mikom aspired to locate inner peace and connect with their mother and grandmother while they are still alive, further realizing the ancestral pain that has led to both of these women having mental health issues. Mikom would like to sit with them and offer them the opportunity to be heard and seen in a compassionate and empathic manner. Mikom believed that this offering would not only tap into their inner resiliency but empower their mother and grandmother to actualize their own resiliency that they likely bestowed to Mikom.

Mikom's one outstanding concern was finding ways to feel safe enough to reduce/eliminate their substance use disorder. We addressed this concern by drawing from the two-eyed seeing approach (Forbes et al., 2020; Marsh et al., 2015), in which Western and Indigenous beliefs would both be used to help Mikom understand specific coping and self-care practices to replace the use of alcohol and drugs to soothe their pain. By means of "Reclaiming Cultural Narratives" (see Figure 3.2), Mikom was enlightened by the ability to deconstruct and externalize shame and guilt, and reauthor their narrative (Semmler & Williams, 2000). In recognizing that their father did not leave because Mikom "was never good enough," they were able to surrender emotions associated with being abandoned and feeling unloved.

By breaking the cycle of intrusive thoughts and not engaging in substance use, Mikom's new narrative included more self-compassion, self-care practices, and forgiveness towards their father and mother for what happened. Mikom stopped feeling responsible for their father's actions and voiced an interest to reintroduce Indigenous healing practices such as teachings from the medicine wheel, smudging, attending sweat lodges, and drumming ceremonies on their former reserve (Ford-Ellis, 2019). Mikom will continue to need time and loving kindness to feel whole again, but these revelations and culturally responsive and Indigenized support will help Mikom and their future generations find long-term healing strategies.

Prem

Prem sought therapy for the following reasons:

1. To develop a sense a belonging in his adopted *pardes* (homeland), regardless of the systemic oppression and barriers he experienced as an immigrant.
2. To overcome the grief and associated trauma of leaving India, his family, and potential life in a culture that is familiar to him.

To begin, Prem was offered psychoeducation and information about intersectionality. Prem listed the more notable social identities within his intersectionality; he identifies as a 90-year-old first-generation South Asian immigrant, 1947 Partition of India/Pakistan survivor, father of three children, retired educator, and heterosexual cisgender male. He reluctantly referred to himself as a Canadian citizen given the mistreatment and barriers he has experienced since he immigrated to Canada in the early 1960s. His perception on citizenship was an ideal segue into understanding how his social identities were ignored and silenced. Prem expressed that he not only experienced colonialism and other forms of oppression in Canada but also in India (Bhatia & Priya, 2021). He added that originating from a poor family stigmatized him and did not offer him the educational prospects for which he yearned. He felt that he had to leave the oppression present in India to actualize his professional aspirations in Canada.

Before migrating to Canada, Prem was under the impression that Canada was a safe, rich, and welcoming country that treated everyone fairly. Initially, his teaching colleagues in northern Alberta proved Prem's beliefs true; however, over the years and at pivotal stages of his career, he was confronted with different forms of racial inequity and discrimination. At the time, he was unable to call these events traumatic, but in retrospect, Prem lived in fear and did not feel safe in several situations due to his intersectionality.

To build on his narrative of internalized oppression and core beliefs, I asked Prem a prompt from Table 8.1, "Life Phases and Social Identity Stages": "What are your reflections regarding your lived experience as an immigrant or BIPOC?" Prem said that this was a very difficult question to answer as he had hoped that previously internalized oppression would have decreased upon arriving in a country as *brilliant* as Canada. He stated that in some ways, he was able to provide a better life for his family and additional academic and career possibilities for his children. He invested time in his children by consistently preserving culture in their household in a very fun, natural, and experiential manner (Sodhi, 2017). He travelled back to India with his wife and offspring numerous times so that his family could stay connected with extended family throughout India. Prem found returning to Canada after these memorable trips difficult as he had to leave elderly relatives and his siblings behind. These guilt-ridden moments still haunt Prem to this day. We discussed the importance of shedding core beliefs of guilt and helplessness and replacing them with strategies to become a productive ally. Prem has always given back to the community and educated others about South Asian culture and the Sikh religion by providing presentations and writing books. He has also shared his narrative of survival with his grandchildren, who continue to learn from his immigrant legacy.

From here, Prem was ready to talk more about the trauma he encountered in India and Canada. He reviewed Table 2.1, "Types of Trauma," and identified the following as forms of trauma that resonated with him: colonial trauma, cultural trauma, developmental trauma, migratory trauma, systemic trauma, racial trauma, collective trauma, and intergenerational trauma. Prem stated that these categories of trauma influenced the person he is today while also stymying him from moving past his father's disciplinary tactics, mother's death, and regrets about immigrating. Each type of trauma overlapped with another during his childhood, adolescence, and adulthood, encouraging him to default to trauma responses. While considering Table 2.1, Prem experienced flashbacks of his childhood. We honoured the somatic responses associated with these flashbacks, particularly locating where the sensations were stored physically in Prem. He indicated that he was feeling sadness and noticed the sensation in his heart. To understand this further, we discussed Figure 3.6, "Culturally Relevant Trauma Responses" and how Prem oscillated between fight, flight, freeze, and fawn. Prem voiced that he was able to demonstrate resiliency throughout his life, whether it was during his academics, interactions with his father, or trying to sustain a bicultural identity in Canada. Prem asserted his career trajectory without support from his father, although he often immersed himself in his profession to distract himself from uncomfortable emotions and overachieved to preclude feeling inadequate. Prem attests that he had the same expectations for his children and grandchildren, whom he asks to "go to the top" and not settle for second best.

There were times where Prem stayed silent when he was berated by his father or internalized familial shame for being compared to other siblings' academic and professional achievements. As a cycle breaker, Prem was able to overcome his people pleasing tendencies and codependency, make decisions based on his value system and the betterment of his future, and balance familial expectations. He is aware of how his past is linked to these trauma responses and understands that certain trauma responses can be conflicting if you belong to a collectivist culture; that is, cultural expectations may be misconstrued for trauma responses. He agreed that some of these expectations are dated and need re-evaluation, and he believes that our conversation illuminated the grief that is consuming him.

We discussed the concept of "Situational Grief" (described in Chapter 3) as an in-between state that is accompanied by non-linear stages of grief. There was a plethora of events in Prem's life that warrant grieving, including his discordant relationship with his father, his mother's passing, and experiencing racial discrimination and loss of family when moving to Canada (Nesteruk, 2018). Prem conceptualized his grief, particularly the death of a loved one, in this manner:

- Received sudden news of the death; he was unaware of the extent of the relative's declining health due to living in another country.
- Experienced powerlessness for not being able to travel abroad to be with family due to age and the COVID-19 pandemic restrictions.
- Revisited existential conditions and reasons for migrating to Canada.
- Questioned his mortality, suggesting that grief is a response to fear of dying.

- Felt excluded from the collective grieving process; he could only support from afar.
- Lacked any form of closure; he only had peripheral involvement in funeral and other cultural/religious ceremonies and rituals.

Using grief journalling prompts, to help Prem move from mourning and regret to memorializing a late family member, I asked him to share his most cherished memory, how he can forgive himself, and how he could demonstrate self-compassion. Prem was able to recall a childhood memory that included his late mother. He is now the only surviving child/sibling. As his mother was Hindu and his father was Sikh, Prem often went to the *Mandhir* (Hindu temple) with his mother. As a child, he felt safe, protected, and held by his mother as he sat in her lap and listened to *bhagans* (religious hymns) sung by the congregation. Afterwards, they would go for a walk around the village, where she would share stories about his maternal grandparents with him. He admits that he was closest to her and started denoucing the patriarchy and South Asian gender roles given his mother's perception of inequality of women in India. When his mother was diagnosed with uterine cancer in 1964, Prem was devastated. He questioned why this was happening. He blamed himself for moving away and not reciprocating the protection his mother provided towards him during his childhood. Fortunately, Prem and his wife were able to visit his mother during the summer of 1966, a few months before she passed away.

Prem understood that holding onto this blame was not healthy and held him back from truly commemorating his mother. He realized that he was not only grieving the loss of his mother but also that of a caring and loving father figure. Grief was indeed complicated, but Prem was ready to let go of the pain that he carried for over 50 years. He did his best over the decades and made multiple trips to India to solidify the bond he had with his family. He started accepting the fact that moving away from India and disconnecting from certain family members was his attempt to protect his sanity and start over. For once, he needed to put his needs first and not succumb to familial expectations or guilt.

By prioritizing his needs, through continuing bonds theory, Prem was able to finally celebrate the influence his mother had on his life and all the lessons she taught him before she passed away. Prem remembers his mother taking in disenfranchised women from the village who were being abused by their spouses. These teachings supported Prem's desire to be a self-proclaimed feminist and stand out as one of the more resourceful, progressive, and approachable "uncles" in his city's South Asian community; he credits his mother for this privilege. Having this role allowed Prem to come to terms with the lack of relationship with his father. He was able to forgive himself for making the choice to immigrate to Canada and absolve his father for being a stern parental figure. He recognized that his father was not capable of being an affectionate person due to his own harsh upbringing. As a result, Prem was determined not to pass this trait down to his children and compassionately became the opposite of his father. He renarrated his childhood with his children and made sure they had the most magical and loving upbringing; this essentially annulled the hardships and racism that Prem experienced upon immigrating to Canada. To feel connected to his culture, he taught his children to be grateful of their heritage and ancestry (Bhugra & Becker, 2005). By witnessing their appreciation for their culture and further preserving that culture in his grandchildren, Prem felt proud and accomplished. Again, he was able to let go of his anxiety and guilt, and through grieving, he was able to accept his decision to migrate to a country that he believed would offer more academic and professional advantages than India.

For the final part of the IHT framework, Prem's Eastern healing practices included "Silencing the Inner Cultural Critic" and "Intersectional Healing." Both techniques are discussed in Chapter 3. Prem reinforced silencing the inner cultural critic by using these strategies: asserting himself in all existing ecosystems, becoming further aware of what activates his nervous system as well as the accompanied somatic feedback, and acknowledging the origins of the inner cultural critic. This final strategy involved identifying whose voice he was listening to and whether the voice was internal or external to him. Prem stated that upon hearing his inner cultural critic, he will remind himself of all the accomplishments he and his wife achieved in Canada, particularly the successes that his children have had in their personal lives, academics, and chosen careers. He refuses to default to trauma responses that would stagnate his progress or devolve into second-guessing his decision to migrate out of India.

As a senior, intersectional healing has played a significant role in helping Prem co-regulate and *heal forward* with family and community members. It has brought diverse South Asian communities together and has reinforced cultural, linguistic, and religious preservation within future generations. Prem spearheaded several endeavours and events (e.g., lecture series, children's gym days, and panel discussions) to ensure that there was continuity in cultural preservation. Together, Prem and other community members were able to break barriers and develop a consistent productive allyship that helped individuals of different generational backgrounds feel welcomed and safe in their adopted homeland. In essence, Prem embraced and exemplified *Chardi Kala* (a Sikh concept meaning "to live in eternal bliss and have a positive mindset", noted in Chapter 3), which has helped him process, unlearn, and heal from the several types of trauma he experienced (Kaur, 2021; Sodhi, 2021a). He said that these practices are reminders of the inner strength and resiliency required to actively partake in collective healing alongside consistent community cultural preservation and togetherness.

Isla

Isla has two intentions for therapy:

1. To unpack and resolve her past trauma and rebuild her future.
2. To forgive her parents and reconnect with family.

After the initial meeting paperwork was reviewed and discussed, Isla was asked what she knew about intersectionality. Isla said that she was not familiar with the word and was intrigued. Psychoeducation and definitions of intersectionality were provided to Isla as well as an opportunity to share her social identities. Isla said she identifies as a 40-year-old Latine, lower class, separated mother of three children, and heterosexual cisgender female. Upon disclosing this information, Isla felt she was being judged. She was reassured that she was in a safe space, as mentioned in the informed consent document, and that everything that is communicated in session is confidential barring certain circumstances (i.e., harm to others, oneself, or children). Isla's main concern was her former husband learning about her attending therapy. She stated that she was still afraid of him and worried that receiving support in therapy would impact the custody of her children. Isla was comforted and reminded that attending therapy would make her a stronger parent to her children. Intrusive thoughts about feeling judged had been ruminating within her from the day she left her husband. She was frequently traumatized by the verbal and physical abuse she received from her in-laws and from not having a husband who would protect her.

We identified oppressive systems that impact her intersectionality: the patriarchy and capitalism. Isla witnessed gender oppression amongst her relatives and experienced it herself during her upbringing in El Salvador (Bell, 2013). She was taught to be subservient to her father and husband and to listen rather than be heard. She was instructed not to ask too many questions and to do what she was told. This left Isla conflicted, as she noticed the intergenerational harm that the patriarchy had inflicted on the matriarchs of her family. In addition to these limitations, capitalism had created barriers for her entrance to the workforce at a mature age. She feels unsupported in establishing her career due to her life stage. While enrolled in business night courses, Isla struggled to be taken seriously by her peers and the owners of the business college alike. She was often referred to as the "older female student," an indicator of her inequality. Isla wanted to withdraw from school on many occasions, but she knew that obtaining an education was integral to her career development. Isla coped in part by envisioning having her own business and independently supporting her children and their aspirations.

I asked Isla a prompt from Table 8.1, "Life Phases and Social Identity Stages": "How did your perceptions of the host country impact cultural preservation in your home environment?" Isla's core beliefs were derived from these perceptions, as she felt inadequate and lacked a sense of belonging due to being excluded and rejected by her in-laws. Isla explained that she had tried to overturn these core beliefs by recalling that her parents and brother helped her to leave a very toxic and stressful in-law arrangement; this event inspired her to consider rebuilding trusting relationships with her family. Isla understood that acceptance, and potentially radical acceptance, could transform her feeling out of place. By letting go of these emotions, Isla was able to authentically transmit culture to her children. These two aspects, re-establishing trust with her family and radical acceptance, almost need to be distinct so that positive cultural traits and healing are intergenerationally passed down (Denov et al., 2019; Tam, 2015).

When presented with Table 2.1, "Types of Trauma," Isla identified with developmental trauma, complex post-traumatic stress disorder (C-PTSD), and systemic trauma. Isla felt constantly unsafe due to living amidst corruption in El Salvador. For Isla, feeling unsafe was compounded by witnessing her uncle being tortured; she regularly trauma responded in the forms of freeze and fawn, and then grounded herself to reconnect with reality. Her post-traumatic stress reaction became post-traumatic stress disorder (PTSD) as Isla had flashbacks and recurrent nightmares of what she had witnessed. Additionally, her marriage at age 17, living with her unsupportive husband and demanding in-laws, her sense of abandonment from her family, grieving her stillborn child, and having an unfaithful spouse who abused drugs left Isla contending with C-PTSD. These events spanned almost 25 years of her life; Isla felt helpless and hopeless about her future. Due to previous feelings of abandonment from her family, she did not know who she could depend upon or trust. Isla's unprocessed trauma resulted in chronic exhaustion, headaches, back pain, and mild paranoia. Isla needed to process her uncle's death and grieve the passing of her stillborn child and challenging marriage.

It was apparent that Isla was interested in becoming self-reliant and feeling safer, which required her to maintain boundaries for herself and children. Isla felt uncomfortable drawing boundaries due to her patriarchal upbringing. Using the "Codependent-Interdependent Spectrum" captured in Figure 3.8, we outlined Isla's attachment style (anxious) and relationship with family. She indicated that her family was quite codependent, enmeshed, and that she had been parentified and involved in role reversal (Arellano et al., 2018). Isla dearly loved her siblings; still, she was often left to take care of them while her parents struggled to manage the hotel. These expectations set a precedent for Isla to be obedient and accommodating to her family's needs before her own. This revelation left Isla feeling conflicted between respecting her parents' intentions and resenting not having been listened to or taken seriously.

Isla was asked what was essential to reconstituting her relationship with her parents and siblings such that it was interdependent rather than codependent. Two words came to Isla's mind: forgiveness and trust. Isla knew that the only way to move forward was to forgive her parents for the choices they had made all through her lifetime and to recognize that their actions were not malicious (Kornfield, 2008). They did not deliberately abandon her; they were following culturally prescribed norms of that time. The accumulation of traumatic events had made this abandonment wound seemingly unhealable. Part of what Isla would like to do in future therapy sessions is explore, process, reframe, grieve, and heal from these traumas, including living in a country where safety is compromised.

To prepare Isla for her reunion with her parents and encourage her to be more assertive, we reviewed the following five guidelines from the "Negotiating Boundaries within a Cultural Space" technique mentioned in Chapter 3:

1. Assess what boundaries looked like; were they respected?
2. Revisit individualist and collectivist values based on situations and events.
3. Consider maintenance protocols; how were boundaries sustained? Were they retracted based on cultural expectations?
4. Reframe and rebuild, nurture, and grow: focus on the present need for flexible boundaries.
5. Offer insight concerning boundary setting and why boundaries need to be established.

This information resonated with Isla and validated her need to stand up for herself towards adverse people and situations in her life. She was able to set small boundaries to increase balance in her life; however, they were never respected, and she was often gaslit. Isla admits that cultural and societal expectations continue to hold her back from maintaining boundaries, as does her fear of offending others (Sodhi, 2008; Tawwab, 2021). She realized that setting and maintaining boundaries require time, energy, and consistent self-confidence. She regularly second-guesses her choice to put her needs first and therefore rescinds her boundary. From this exercise, Isla learned to continue developing patience with herself and others, and to recognize that her rights, time, and visions matter.

Following this exercise, Isla determined that she was ready to examine her internalized grief. We started unpacking the loss of her stillborn child and the lack of support she received at the time of the birth. Originating from a family of seven, Isla always envisioned having five children after attending school and starting a career in business. She felt blessed with her three children and elated when she found out she was pregnant again with her fourth child. She believed that the stress of the toxic in-law interactions and hostile marriage provoked the loss of this child. What scarred her the most was her husband's refusal to have more children with her, who Isla realizes in hindsight was not as invested in the marriage. Over the years, Isla spoke to her unborn baby at night and would apologize to her for not being able to keep her alive. She felt remorseful for what happened. I asked her if she felt comfortable trying other ways of cherishing her baby's memory. Isla said that while she was pregnant, she made a traditional El Salvadorian quilt that she had hoped to swaddle the baby in. After this birth trauma, Isla put the blanket away in her trunk of sentimental belongings. I asked her how she would feel if she brought the blanket out and placed it on the chair next to her bed as a reminder of her unconditional love for the baby. I wondered if this could help her shift from being apologetic to forgiving herself for her loss. We talked about demonstrating self-compassion and untangling the stillbirth from Isla's inability to stay in the marriage. Different forms of grief still intersect for Isla, and she still copes with feeling responsible for all these losses.

To reconcile with these misfortunes, we thought of ways for Isla to feel connected with the person she was before her marriage. She was very proud of her family's determination and resiliency and their ability to pass these values to their children. As the eldest child, Isla felt accountable for being a positive role model for her siblings and had therefore put her identity development aside. As a person who experienced layers of trauma, it would be problematic for Isla to self-forgive. Isla was asked again to separate the root of her suffering from the emotions associated with her grief, as they may be interconnected. By holding onto anger and resentment, she would not be able to let go of the sadness from her past and the decisions her parents made on her behalf. Isla was able to externalize her anger and resentment and understand the need to forgive herself and continue healing.

For the last part of this IHT process, I provided Isla with Table 3.1, "Grounding Techniques, Glimmers, and Self-Soothing Exercises" to help her regulate and heal from these traumas (Dana, 2021). I asked Isla to create a list and integrate content from Table 3.1. For grounding techniques, Isla chose breathwork, having a glass of water, cherishing and holding a safe grounding object. For glimmers, Isla wrote down connecting with nature, watching a sunset, and receiving hugs from her children. Lastly, to self-soothe, Isla enumerated eating favourite foods, relaxing to calming music, and resting. Isla was asked to refer to this list anytime she felt activated or was unable to cope in any situation or interaction.

To conclude, Isla was introduced to the "Trauma-Healing Continuum" (see Figure 3.3) as a starting point for unpacking traumatic events (i.e., gang violence, loss of a child) and how they dysregulated her nervous system and instigated other familial events. Isla also explored the stages of grief (e.g., shock, denial) she experienced, reasons for breaking the intergenerational cycle by attending therapy, participated in grounding and reframing, learned the importance of growth and patience with the healing process, and eventually moved towards some elements of acceptance. Isla is aware that this trauma-healing continuum is non-linear; however, she has the tools now to make sense of the traumas she experienced and to mitigate their impacts.

Yin

Yin's therapeutic aspirations are as follows:

1. To confront the traumas she has experienced throughout her lifetime.
2. To challenge racial barriers and unlearn the model minority myth.

Yin specified that she tried accessing therapy in the past; however, she only attended a handful of free consultations to determine client-therapist compatibility. Although reluctant to engage with a counsellor in the past, Yin was ready to talk more about her history and how it has influenced her current frame of mind. She wanted to process trauma so that she could actualize her potential. We began therapy by introducing psychoeducation and information about intersectionality and its relationship with the associated oppressive systems. Yin itemized her social identities. Yin identifies as a 34-year-old second-generation Chinese immigrant, professor at an American university, and heterosexual cisgender female. She is not married, nor does she have any children. Yin's sexual assault at the age of 11 left a traumatic and lifelong mark on her. She felt judged by extended family members for her lack of traditional social identities as wife and mother and is hassled about "finding" the right person, "settling down," and having children. Yin stated that she has no desire to marry nor have children at this time as she can hardly manage her own matters.

Yin continues to face systemic oppression due to stigma related to her cultural/ethnic/racial background. She has experienced an array of racial inequities, racism, and discrimination throughout her schooling and even within her faculty. She has encountered microaggressions for being hard working and having a strong sense of professionalism, both of which are stereotypes associated with the model minority myth (Yi et al., 2023). Yin internalized this racism and has tried to assimilate more into the host culture by not speaking Cantonese and choosing not to associate with other Chinese professors on campus (Pyke, 2010). She would assert herself towards her colleagues but still feels silenced by members of the host culture. She thought that if she distanced herself from her ancestral culture, she would be able to let go of the model minority myth persona. This was not the case.

Yin was impacted by the significant increase in anti-Asian racism sparked by the COVID-19 pandemic. She experienced hate crime threats from ignorant individuals who believed her family in China was involved in the spread of the virus. She spent a number of months indoors during the pandemic, hoping that such assumptions would be disproven and that she would be able to leave home without fearing for her wellbeing (Choi, 2021). She often reiterated her parents' rationale for migrating to the United States and how her family needed to rebuild their life after experiencing trauma in China. She praises her parents for making this very difficult decision and speaks of how imperative it was for them to offer stability and opportunities to her and her brother. The pandemic became a time for Yin to remind herself of the beauty of her cultural background and to create a positive association with her ethnicity. This would hopefully culminate in acquired self-compassion for how she was treated throughout her lifetime for being Asian.

I posed the following prompt from Table 8.1, "Life Phases and Social Identity Stages," to Yin: "What is your recollection of the cultural/ethnic/racial breakdown of your peer/school group?" This inquiry caused Yin to dissociate for a moment until she grounded herself with a *Yuan*, a special Chinese coin given to her by her late aunt. We talked about what transpired when she dissociated, and what she felt somatically. While attending to some discomfort in her throat, Yin said that she was reminded of a time when she felt unworthy and inadequate in her school; she shared core beliefs that show up when she is not heard and seen by her colleagues during staff meetings. In China, children between the ages of three to six enroll in full-day kindergarten from 8am to 5pm; hers was highly structured with strict disciplining for not listening or completing homework. At the end of the kindergarten program, students are required to complete a final examination to graduate to primary school. Yin was thankful that she moved to the United States at age five years and missed taking the final examination.

Yin said that her peer/school group in China was homogeneous except for the occasional diplomat's child. She appreciated spending time with her Chinese classmates who originated from her family's village. She said that her kindergarten program emphasized Chinese language, arts, music, and values which she believes influenced her ethnic identity formation. This helped Yin to solidify her cultural values and beliefs when she arrived in the United States and there were limited cultural resources in New Jersey. Yin tried to maintain this mindset, but her classes were mostly populated with white students. This further reinforced her model minority myth, the years of microaggressions, and affiliated racial trauma that followed. We discussed the meaning of externalizing core beliefs of unworthiness and feelings of inadequacy and replacing them with moments of cultural empowerment.

Yin read Table 2.1, "Types of Trauma," and pointed to cultural trauma, developmental trauma, migratory trauma, systemic trauma, racial trauma, collective trauma, and intergenerational trauma as wounds she carried. Yin's trauma started at age one with the death of her paternal aunt in the 1989 *Tiananmen Square* Protests and Massacre. Due to the shock surrounding this event, her family did not grieve or heal from this tragic event and passed down their unresolved cultural trauma to Yin and her older brother. To this day, she believes her parents and grandparents feel immense guilt and have modelled staying busy and occupied to distract oneself from sadness. We reviewed the "Culturally Relevant Trauma Responses" (Figure 3.7) to learn more about how Yin copes in her everyday life. She stated that she gravitates towards the flight and fawn responses, depending on the situation. She was encouraged by her family to be academically motivated, professionally focussed, and an overachiever in all realms of her life while simultaneously people pleasing and being codependent, and highly influenced by family when making decisions about her life. These qualities along with her trauma responses reinforced the model minority myth. In our conversation about these trauma responses, we explored whether she was indeed experiencing a trauma response or if these were cultural and/ or societal expectations placed upon her. This is differentiated based upon how it activates her core beliefs and the expectations that were modelled by family members. Yin confirmed that it was a combination of both and wanting to reinvent herself to become more assertive in designated personal and professional spaces.

This led to the conversation about "ethnic guilt" and her wish to be a cycle breaker. As noted in Chapter 3, ethnic guilt is comprised of:

- A fear of offending
- People pleasing tendencies
- Needing to compromise excessively
- Sacrificing inner happiness
- Experiencing feelings of inadequacy

Yin saw herself reflected in this description of ethnic guilt and noticed that she learned these tendencies from her conflict avoidant mother and grandmother. During her life, they reminded Yin of the importance of compliance and agreeability, even if what others said made Yin uncomfortable. Yin felt she did not have the choice to express how she truly felt about her family's trauma or her own. She was worried about offending elders, teachers, and friends and therefore overcompensated for her actions. In the end, she put others' happiness before her own and maintained this people pleasing cycle by believing her needs were not as important.

I asked Yin how she envisioned breaking this cycle, and she responded that her first step would be to trust that her needs matter and to become more assertive. She would begin by addressing her concerns to her family who were desperate to see her married and have children. She would be honest with them about her plans for her future, which would include adjusting society's perceptions about Chinese culture and immigrants rather than becoming a wife and mother. Yin aspires to embrace her cultural background and help eliminate anti-Asian racism through either teaching or community work (Byon et al., 2022; Gover et al., 2020). Yin also hopes to voice how she feels within her faculty, stop agreeing to teach more courses, and instead start an Asian Graduate Students Association. She believes taking these actions will help establish better boundaries and more respect with her colleagues who occasionally expect her to compromise too much and disregard her needs.

Yin's previous reflections about ethnic guilt and cycle breaking prepared her to explore grief. Yin had been erratically connected to her Chinese culture for many years. She yearned to reconnect with her heritage and spend quality time – with her parents, brother, grandparents, and extended family on her terms. She respects her family's ability to rebuild their life after experiencing trauma in China. She would like to learn more about her ancestors that lived in China and some of the customs and rituals that were lost upon migrating to the United States. She hopes that these interactions will counterbalance the stigma related to being Asian and help her develop more appreciation for her cultural background. Yin would like to grieve the migratory obstacles that presented upon arrival to the United States; she had already carried the racism and trauma with her for over 25 years before the hate crime. She reminded herself of her cultural pride before leaving China and the necessity of reconnecting with Chinese peers who have similar values.

We explored the Four Noble Truths from Buddhist psychology to understand and abdicate suffering from Yin's life. The Four Noble Truths are Dukkha (suffering); the origins of suffering; the liberation from suffering; and the path that ends suffering (Neimeyer & Young-Eisendrath, 2015; Tirch et al., 2016). Yin disclosed that the main suffering consisting of racism and trauma experienced throughout her lifetime. The origins of both varied; however, the intergenerational and migratory components were notable and left an imprint on her intersectionality. She believes that she will be able to liberate herself from both forms of suffering via productive allyship in the community and rediscovering her culture through more boundaried family interactions. To maintain her feeling of liberation, Yin plans on writing a book about her lived experience so that future generations can learn about her struggles as a second-generation Chinese woman who survived the COVID-19 pandemic.

For the last part of IHT framework, derived from Chapter 3, Yin was asked to create a "Cultural Safety Road Map." This plan consisted of comparing Yin's original road map or narrative with the renarrated version of this road map that included grounding techniques, desensitization, and healing strategies. Yin was able to share her original narrative in Part 3 by discussing events related to personal and racial trauma. Yin said that when she experienced intrusive trauma-related thoughts or somatic feedback, she practiced more meditative techniques or body scans to ground herself. As mentioned earlier in her treatment plan, she carries a Chinese coin that her aunt gave her; this coin helps her ground in spaces that are not conducive to meditation or body scans. Yin is unlearning default people pleasing and replacing these tendencies with being assertive and drawing boundaries. She is augmenting her safety by creating productive allyships that will teach members of the host culture about Chinese culture while also demystifying stereotypes (Akbar, 2020). When she experiences somatic feedback, she takes a step back and reminds herself of the cycles she has broken and the barriers she has overcome. This segment of the IHT process allowed Yin to take agency, make critical life decisions, and create a path towards her long-term wellbeing.

To solidify Yin's healing, we reviewed "Intersectional Healing" as conveyed in Chapter 3. Yin would like to overcome her model minority myth, educate others, and dismantle white supremacy by rallying and healing together. I encouraged Yin to locate self-regulation/grounding techniques, but I also recognize that intersectional healing requires co-regulation with community and like-minded individuals. Yin would like to preserve culture within herself and transmit it towards her students, nieces, and nephews. Yin has been able to organize events in her community that vibrantly celebrate Chinese culture. She was elated to see the generational and cultural span of people who attended and learned about these occasions. Within her classroom, she implemented more culturally responsive and trauma-informed teaching strategies (Gay, 2018; Samuels, 2018), which helped decentre colonial and eurocentric beliefs and perceptions about Chinese culture. These initiatives helped Yin to break barriers, be more proactive about sharing her culture, and generate more allyship and cultural awareness in academia.

Part 5 highlights and provides discourse about embodying healing through community and self-care practices.

References

Akbar, M. (2020). *Beyond ally: The pursuit to racial justice*. Publish Your Purpose Press.

Arellano, B., Mier-Chairez, J., Tomek, S., & Hooper, L. M. (2018). Parentification and language brokering: An exploratory study of the similarities and differences in their relations to continuous and dichotomous mental health outcomes. *Journal of Mental Health Counseling*, 40(4), 353–373.

Bell, O. (2013). Poverty and gender inequality in post-war El Salvador. *Global Majority E-Journal*, 4(1), 27–39.

Bhatia, S., & Priya, K. R. (2021). Coloniality and psychology: From silencing to re-centering marginalized voices in postcolonial times. *Review of General Psychology*, 25(4), 422–436.

Bhugra, D., & Becker, M. (2005). Migration, cultural bereavement and cultural identity. *World Psychiatry: Official Journal of the World Psychiatric Association*, 4(1), 18–24.

Bowlby, J. (1988). *A secure base: Parent-child attachment and healthy human development*. Basic Books.

Byon, A. H., Preston, D. C., Assalone, A. E., & Elliott, K. C. (2022). The role of advocacy organizations in student activism: Black lives matter and stop anti-Asian hate. *New Directions for Student Services*, 2022(180), 71–81.

Choi, S. (2021). "People look at me like I am the virus": Fear, stigma, and discrimination during the COVID-19 pandemic. *Qualitative Social Work*, 20(1–2), 233–239.

Dana, D. (2018). *The polyvagal theory in therapy: Engaging the rhythm of regulation*. W.W. Norton.

Dana, D. (2021). *Anchored: How to befriend your nervous system using polyvagal theory*. Sound True.

Denov, M., Fennig, M., Rabiau, M. A., & Shevell, M. C. (2019). Intergenerational resilience in families affected by war, displacement, and migration: "It runs in the family". *Journal of Family Social Work*, 22(1), 17–45.

Forbes, A., Ritchie, S. D., Walker, J., & Young, N. L. (2020). Applications of two-eyed seeing in primary research focused on Indigenous health: A scoping review. *International Journal of Qualitative Methods*, 19, 1–18.

Ford-Ellis, A. G. (2019). How is the medicine wheel considered in therapeutic practice? *Journal of Concurrent Disorders*, 1(3), 78–93.

Gay, G. (2018). *Culturally responsive teaching: Theory, research and* practice (3rd ed.). Teachers College Press.

Goffman, E. (1963). *Stigma: Notes on the management of spoiled identity*. Simon & Schuster.

Gover, A. R., Harper, S. B., & Langton, L. (2020). Anti-Asian hate crime during the COVID-19 pandemic: Exploring the reproduction of inequality. *American Journal of Criminal Justice*, 45(4), 647–667.

Heller, D. P. (2019). *The power of attachment: How to create deep and lasting intimate relationships*. Sounds True.

John, S. E., & Segal, D. L. (2015). Case conceptualization. In R. L. Cautin & S. O. Lilienfeld (Eds.), *The encyclopedia of clinical psychology* (pp. 1–4). John Wiley and Sons.

Kaur, V. (2021). *See no stranger: A memoir and manifesto of revolutionary love*. One World.

Kilcullen, M. L., & Day, A. (2018). Culturally informed case conceptualisation: Developing a clinical psychology approach to treatment planning for non-Indigenous psychologists working with Aboriginal and Torres Strait Islander clients. *Clinical Psychologist, 22,* 280–289.

Kornfield, J. (2008). *The art of forgiveness, lovingkindness, and peace.* W.W. Norton.

Marsh, T. N., Coholic, D., Cote-Meek, S., & Najavits, L. M. (2015). Blending Aboriginal and western healing methods to treat intergenerational trauma with substance use disorder in Aboriginal peoples who live in Northeastern Ontario, Canada. *Harm Reduction Journal, 12*(14), 1–12.

Monteiro, L. M., Musten, R. F., & Compson, J. (2017). Traditional and contemporary mindfulness: Finding the middle path in the tangle of concerns. In B. A. Gaudiano (Ed.), *Mindfulness: The roots of mindfulness: History, philosophy, and definitions* (pp. 239–262). Routledge.

Neimeyer, R. A., & Young-Eisendrath, P. (2015). Assessing a Buddhist treatment for bereavement and loss: The mustard seed project. *Death Studies, 39*(5), 263–273.

Nesteruk, O. (2018). Immigrants coping with transnational deaths and bereavement: The influence of migratory loss and anticipatory grief. *Family Process, 57*(4), 1012–1028.

Paré, D. A. (2013). *The practice of collaborative counselling and psychotherapy: Developing skills in culturally mindful helping.* SAGE Publications.

Porges, S. W. (2011). *The polyvagal theory: Neurophysiological foundations of emotions, attachment, communication, and self-regulation.* W.W. Norton & Co.

Pyke, K. D. (2010). What is internalized racial oppression and why don't we study it? Acknowledging racism's hidden injuries. *Sociological Perspectives, 53,* 551–572.

Rogers, C. R. (1961). *On becoming a person.* Houghton Mifflin Company.

Rogers, C. R. (1989). Client-centered therapy. In H. Kirschenbaum & V. L. Henderson (Eds.), *Carl Rogers: Dialogues* (pp. 9–40). Houghton Mifflin Company.

Samuels, A. J. (2018). Exploring culturally responsive pedagogy: Teachers' perspectives on fostering equitable and inclusive classrooms. *SRATE Journal, 21*(1), 22–30.

Semmler, P. L., & Williams, C. B. (2000). Narrative therapy: A storied context for multicultural counselling. *Journal of Multicultural Counseling and Development, 28*(1), 51–61.

Sodhi, P. K. (2008). Bicultural identity formation of second-generation Indo-Canadians. *Canadian Ethnic Studies, 40*(2), 187–199.

Sodhi, P. K. (2017). *Exploring immigrant and sexual minority mental health: Reconsidering multiculturalism.* Routledge.

Sodhi, P. K. (2021a). The Sikh spirit of Chardi Kala (resilience) as a cure for grief. Panelist. *Parliament of the World's Religions virtual conference,* October 16–18, 2021.

Sodhi, P. K. (2021b). Decolonizing psychotherapeutic practices for BIPOC clients. Webinar hosted by the *Canadian Counselling and Psychotherapy Association,* October 27, 2021.

Sperry, L., & Sperry, J. (2012). *Case conceptualization.* Taylor & Francis.

Sperry, L., & Sperry, J. (2020). *Case conceptualization: Mastering this competency with ease and confidence* (2nd ed.). Routledge.

Tam, K.-P. (2015). Understanding intergenerational cultural transmission through the role of perceived norms. *Journal of Cross-Cultural Psychology, 46*(10), 1260–1266.

Tawwab, N. G. (2021). *Set boundaries, find peace: A guide to reclaiming yourself.* TarcherPerigee.

Thich, N. H. (1999). *The heart of the Buddha' teaching: Transforming suffering into peace, joy, and liberation.* Broadway Books.

Tirch, D., Siberstein, L. R., & Kolts, R. L. (2016). *Buddhist psychology and cognitive-behavioral therapy.* The Guilford Press.

Yi, J., La, R., Lee, B. A., & Saw, A. (2023). Internalization of the model minority myth and sociodemographic factors shaping Asians/Asian Americans' experiences of discrimination during COVID-19. *American Journal of Community Psychology, 71*(1–2), 123–135.

Part 5

Concluding Thoughts and Offerings

Concluding Thoughts and Offerings

Chapter 10

Embodying Healing Through Community and Self-Care

The late bell hooks challenged systems associated with white supremist capitalist patriarchy; she attested, "If we want a beloved community, we must stand for justice, have recognition for difference without attaching difference to privilege" (hooks, 1993, p. 10). Building upon her words, consistent allyship both inside and outside of therapeutic practice requires individuals and communities to collaborate, voice solidarity, and apply learned knowledge into practice. Coming full circle, and signifying how racism can shape the psyche of a child to becoming a young adult, I would like to share (with her permission) a statement of intent written by my daughter for her university application:

> *It was not until I experienced racism first-hand that I realized children often let their ignorance supersede their humility. As a third-generation South Asian immigrant who was born and raised in Canada, I undoubtedly became naively comfortable surrounding myself with mostly white people. When I was eight-years-old, I met Grace; she was a green-eyed, blonde-haired girl, and we instantly became best friends. One day, Grace mentioned that she was approached by another girl in our class; she was asked why she became friends with me specifically because I was Indian. This certainly did not influence Grace or her opinion of me, but I was left confused and crushed. My eight-year-old self was questioning why it mattered what culture or race I was, and why it would affect my friendships. It opened my eyes to the internalized racism that could be found everywhere and changed my worldview. I was no longer oblivious to the fact that I looked different from my classmates.*
>
> *Several years of unlearning were needed for me to heal from the shame I experienced anytime my cultural background was discussed. My parents made tremendous efforts to encourage involvement with the local Punjabi community. I was enrolled in language, religion, and dance classes; yet what I soon realized is that I felt excluded and in fact somewhat out of place as I was not "Punjabi" enough. I literally belonged to two different worlds and did not feel like a part of either of them.*

DOI: 10.4324/9781003216568-16

The racist comment that was made to my best friend almost ten years ago awakened me. With time, I am able to live in both cultures and no longer feeling shameful of my Punjabi heritage. Rather, I am educating my peers on internalized racism and how to eliminate it. When I put everything into perspective, I am thankful that Grace was approached, allowing me to better understand the issues people of colour confront on a daily basis. Now, I can live authentically in both worlds.

One of the aspirations of this book is to represent how to evolve from being culturally competent to trauma-informed and anti-racist practitioners by decolonizing therapeutic and academic spaces. This can and will transpire by dismantling systems of oppression and replacing these systems with more culturally responsive and Eastern healing practices. With intentionality, I am offering the decolonized mental health framework and inclusion and healing therapy (IHT) framework discussed in Chapter 8 to meet the need for therapists to provide more Eastern-style care to BIPOC communities. The five-section IHT model (the steps of which are as follows: exploring intersectionality, recognizing encounters with systemic oppression, processing unresolved trauma, relinquishing suffering, and applying Eastern healing practices) is used in Part 4 to exemplify its efficacy with the intergenerational BIPOC narratives. The key takeaway from Part 4 is that everyone's narrative carries an abundance of pain that deserves personalized and culturally responsive attention to support the healing process.

Healing of this calibre entails distinguishing between and attending to community care and self-care. Community or collective care suggests holding others accountable, sharing resources, watching over and connecting with others, being involved in one's community, having access to community support, feeling grounded in one's community, and engaging in like-minded support systems. In contrast, self-care features rest, socializing, nutrition, movement, self-development, and setting boundaries. What might work for an individual may not necessarily work for a collectivist community; thus, individuals may need to focus on amplifying critical, restorative, and liberation-related therapeutic work (Harro, 2000). Self-care for individual BIPOC may go against the grain of the collective.

Several items outlined in Singh et al.'s (2020) article are foundational to decolonizing therapy. Some such constructs are critical race theory, liberational psychology, and intersectionality. Essentially, by subscribing to these theories, we challenge positions of power and colonial influences within counselling and academic settings. Critical race theory (Delgado & Stefancic, 2017) and intersectional theory (Crenshaw, 1989, 1991) are addressed in Chapter 4; however, anti-oppressive frameworks such as liberation psychology (Burton & Guzzo, 2020; Martín-Baró, 1996) and Harro's Cycle of Liberation (2000) are found within this chapter.

Like Freire's work (1970), liberation psychology's purpose is to empower and heal the oppressed individual, reflect upon their ancestors' victories, transform self-perception, and create change to relinquish suffering from one's life (Comas-Díaz & Torres Rivera, 2020). Liberation psychology was developed based on the scarcity of social justice and Eastern perspectives within Western psychological practices. Created by Ignacio Martín-Baró (1996), he stated that:

> Liberation psychology would take up the perspectives of the oppressed and support those who experience oppression to reclaim their histories, resist socio-political structures that sought to oppress them, and use cultural methods from their ancestors to organize and strengthen their cultures and traditions.
>
> (cited in Singh et al., 2020, p. 266;
> Chavez et al., 2016)

Liberation psychologists advocate for sociopolitical justice and the admonition of systemic oppression; they believe that regardless of intersectionality, individuals can globally survive and decentre oppression (Comas-Díaz & Torres Rivera, 2020). Practitioners that subscribe to liberation psychology empower their clients by augmenting their inner strength and resilience. Liberation psychology is considered a decolonized approach that eschews individualist and eurocentric psychotherapeutic values and beliefs (Burton & Gómez, 2015) and adopts a more restorative and collective care approach to healing.

If we revisit Harro's work (2000) with liberation of individuals, communities, and society in mind, we can discern the steps to understanding personalized trauma and consequently transform feeling liberated into a healing practice. As conveyed by Ratts et al. (2015), graduate students are encouraged to explore each client's narrative at intrapersonal, interpersonal, institutional, community, public policy, and international/global levels and therefore integrate this information into treatment plans. Similarly, Goodman et al. (2004) states that counselling psychology graduate students should broaden their perspective across three levels: (a) the *macro* level: government, policy, and social norms; (b) the *meso* level: community and organization; and (c) the *micro* level: individual and families, to completely appreciate culturally responsive and social justice work. These are both examples of how practitioners may be trained to incorporate tenets of liberation psychology into their clinical work.

Respectively, in a decolonized context and to borrow from Gabor Maté's wise sentiments, "all of Western medicine is built on getting rid of pain, which is not the same as healing. Healing is the capacity to hold pain" (Maté, 2004). Within several oppressive systems, communities continue to hold intergenerational pain while simultaneously trying to heal from trauma.

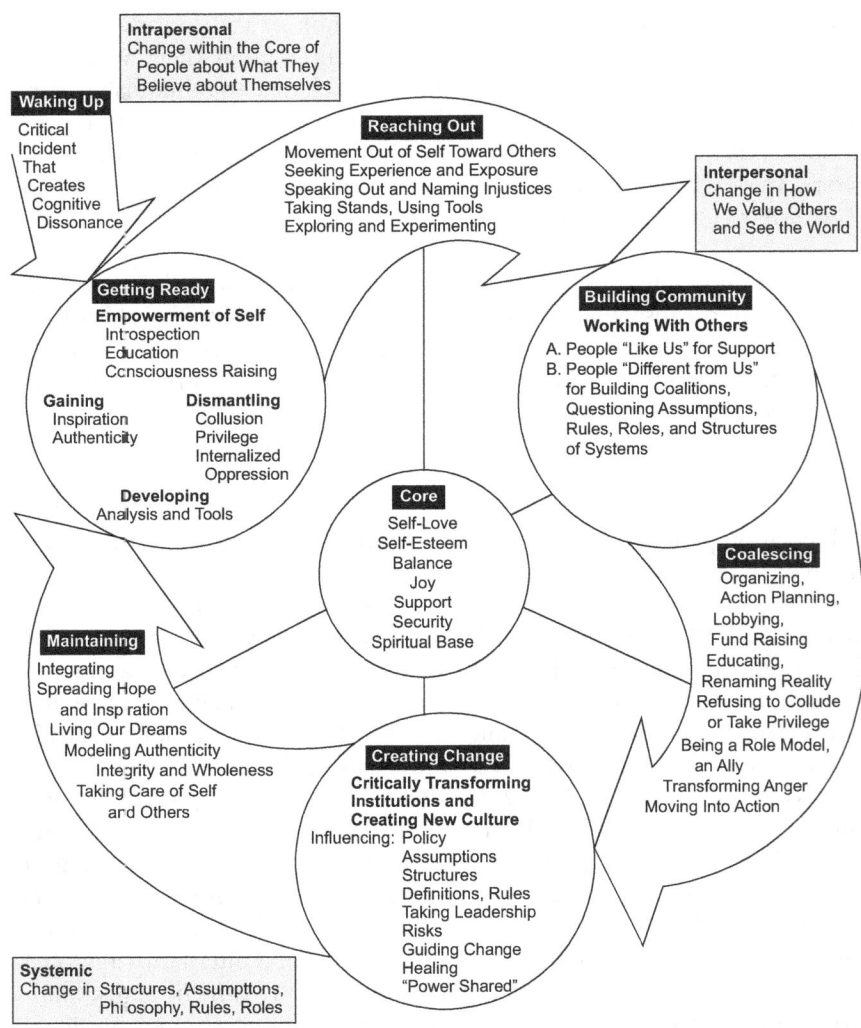

Figure 10.1 The cycle of liberation (Harro, 2000) – with permission from Taylor and Francis

Individuals could start this process of holding pain at the meso level to foster community/collective care and long-standing camaraderie.

Figure 10.1 illustrates how liberation can transpire and pain can be renounced. Here is a thicker description of each component of this model:

1. The *Core*: attributes that bring cohesiveness to the overall cycle of liberation. According to Harro (2013), liberation is the "practice of love,

finding balance, development of competence, belief that one can succeed, not being alone, commitment to change, and lastly passion and
compassion" (p. 469). These qualities set a peaceful and collective tone
for the remainder of this model.

2. *Waking Up*: becoming aware of a traumatic event (e.g., collective
   trauma) that causes inner turmoil, disconnect from the world, and an
   urgency to become woke.
3. *Getting Ready*: recognizing inner resources (e.g., educational privileges,
   tools), exploring options to dismantle harmful oppressive systems and
   groupthink, and engaging in more empowering endeavours.
4. *Reaching Out*: having one's voice heard; also accepting that a collective
   effort requests collaboration and crowdsourcing ways to silence oppressive systems that are manifested in our society.
5. *Building Community*: rallying with other like-minded individuals who
   have the same aspirations and visions surrounding an oppression-free
   landscape.
6. *Coalescing*: putting theory or conversations into action by means of
   organizing, collective planning, protests, or productive allyship to reinforce and shift from anger to hopefulness.
7. *Creating Change*: building upon coalescing by emphasizing change with
   official policies, new rules, and anti-oppressive systems. Critical transformation is foundational within this phase.
8. *Maintaining*: allies fortify, improve, and nurture a safe, trusting space and
   work together to amplify and uphold previous collective and urgent work.

Both Harro's (2000) model and liberation psychology respect and acknowledge BIPOC by offering the gradual inclusion of more decolonized
practices in predominantly Western spaces while decentring oppressive
systems. As noted in previous chapters, liberation and anti-oppressive work
can transcend into psychotherapy and social justice spaces in the form
of decolonized and culturally responsive approaches to fieldwork (Singh
et al., 2020). In this book, strategies to identify privilege, abolish power
dynamics, promote cultural safety, and feature decolonized ways of providing psychotherapy to BIPOC clients are highlighted (Dekker, 2016; Tyler, 2021). It strongly underscores how culturally responsive approaches
to therapy can be taught to future mental health practitioners and allies.
Opportunities to work with intersectional clients and their cultural narratives in practicum settings should be encouraged in counsellor training
programs (Sodhi, 2017).

In academia, decolonization "is the channel for generating a postcolonial
education system in Canada and disrupting those normalized discourses
and singularities and allowing diverse voices and perspectives and objectives into 'mainstream' schooling" (Battiste, 2013, p. 107; Reyes et al.,

2021). This perspective can be easily accompanied by Indigenous or feminist pedagogy that supports trauma-informed, anti-oppressive, anti-heteronormative, anti-racist, and culturally responsive teachings and curricula that undeniably create a culture of inclusion.

Respectively, Samuels' (2018) work espouses culturally responsive pedagogy in supporting equitable and inclusive classrooms. She posits that:

> Culturally responsive pedagogy is a student-centered approach to teaching that includes cultural references and recognizes the importance of students' cultural backgrounds and experiences in all aspects of learning. The approach is meant to promote engagement, enrichment, and achievement of all students by embracing a wealth of diversity, identifying and nurturing students' cultural strengths, and validating students' lived experiences and their place in the world.
>
> (pp. 22–23)

Crediting Geneva Gay (2010, 2013), culturally responsive teaching allows educators to create "meaningful connections" with their multicultural learners. There are five essential elements of culturally responsive teaching (Gay, 2002, p. 106):

1. Communicating with ethnically diverse students.
2. Demonstrating caring and building learning communities.
3. Developing a knowledge base about cultural diversity.
4. Including ethnic and cultural diversity content in the curriculum.
5. Responding to ethnic diversity in the delivery of instruction.

Complementing Samuels' (2018) and Gay's (2018) work, I presented research about "Working with and Supporting Multicultural Learners" at the 2019 Algonquin College *Kaleidoscope* Conference and shared a framework (Figure 10.2) detailing how to design an inclusive classroom atmosphere. Figure 10.2 is comprised of the following components (ovals):

Developing an Authentic Presence

- Promote cultural responsiveness; self-reflection about one's cultural background and personal experiences with diversity.
- Challenge cultural assumptions and unpack assumptions/biases.
- Explore personal intersectionality (e.g., culture, ethnicity, race, religion/faith, spirituality, language, gender, gender identity, social class, sexual orientation, ability, education, and age).
- Exemplify humanistic attributes: being non-judgmental, transparent, congruent, and genuine (Rogers, 1961).

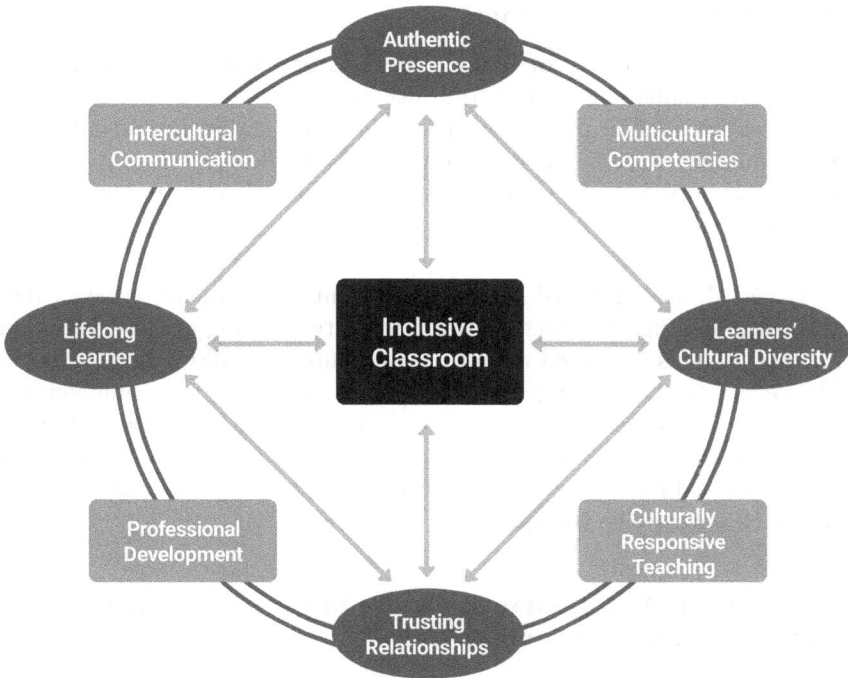

Figure 10.2 Cultivating an inclusive classroom environment (Sodhi, 2019)

Learners' Cultural Diversity

- Acknowledge classroom cultural diversity by creating a welcoming setting; provide guidelines/suggestions for a positive and equitable classroom environment on the first day of class.
- Demonstrate awareness regarding the learners' narrative and intersectionality (Bešić, 2020).
- Become familiar with the learners' lived experience (at home, academic setting, community, and host culture).
- Understand how learning takes place in different cultures; decolonize lesson plans (within assignments, video clips, in-class exercises, etc.).

Building Trusting Relationships

- Create a safe space/classroom culture of inclusion and sense of belonging.
- Engage in active listening regarding multicultural learners' academic needs.
- Appreciate learners' names and pronounce them properly.
- Cultivate a safe academic space to improve learning, self-confidence, and trust in the process.

Becoming Lifelong Learners

- Curate a community of lifelong learners (students and educators) to improve academic retention and success.
- Foster cross-cultural relationships and intercultural communication.
- Encourage learners to collaborate with their fellow peers.
- Provide opportunities for learners to connect and celebrate each other's cultural backgrounds.

The ovals in Figure 10.2 represent the intersecting components (i.e., authentic presence, learners' cultural diversity, trusting relationships, and lifelong learners) required to nurture and support multicultural learners. The rectangles characterize the actions (i.e., multicultural competencies, culturally responsive teaching, professional development, and intercultural communication) that will continuously inspire an inclusive classroom environment. All parts of this framework unite for long-term and consistent cultural awareness to transpire.

As we conclude this chapter, these progressive future directions should be noted:

- Anti-racism and decolonization require deep and substantial processes of unlearning and relearning.
- Move away from culturally competent philosophies such as awareness, knowledge, and skills and become well versed in more trauma-informed and anti-racist practices.
- Provide dynamic and mandatory courses in culturally responsive pedagogy and competencies (Gay, 2018).
- Offer further professional development trainings/workshops/conferences regarding BIPOC issues and culturally responsive classroom practices (Sodhi, 2017).
- Enhance academic settings with culturally affirming policies, curricula mapping, and teaching practices to decentre systemic oppression. School curricula should include and centre diversity, anti-racism, and decolonization.
- Advocate for mental health and the importance of sharing narratives and vulnerability.
- Create inclusive and intersectional mental health resources.

The main focus for writing this book is to share decolonized, culturally responsive, and trauma-informed therapeutic strategies for BIPOC communities. Techniques are provided to empower the reader, break intergenerational cycles, and therefore facilitate healing from past trauma. As a society, we must embrace the importance of learning as a community as it is a collaborative process. We are further connected because of numerous social media platforms; news travels fast, more than ever before. A book, webinar, or presentation will only educate you so far; it is essential to attend trainings and cultural events to capture the nuances associated with the BIPOC community.

I would be remiss for not highlighting that becoming trauma-informed, anti-racist, decolonized practitioners is a lifelong learning process strengthened by attentive listening to BIPOC narratives and stories. While writing this book, I have been reflecting upon the solidarity experienced within diverse in-person and virtual platforms. We as BIPOC have collectively voiced our concerns, engaged in knowledge mobilization about a multitude of causes, campaigned movements, and endorsed a growth mindset within society and beyond. This chapter starts with bell hooks' wisdom and now concludes with her wise words: "Solidarity requires sustained, ongoing commitment" (hooks, 2000, p. 67). This can be supported by elevating voices and representing a consistent and productive allyship.

References

Battiste, M. (2013). *Decolonizing education: Nourishing the learning spirit.* Purich.

Bešić, E. (2020). Intersectionality: A pathway towards inclusive education? *Prospects, 49,* 111–122.

Burton, M., & Gómez, L. (2015). Liberation psychology. In I. Parker (Ed.), *Handbook of critical psychology*. Routledge.

Burton, M., & Guzzo, R. (2020). Liberation psychology: Origins and development. In L. Comas-Díaz & E. Torres Rivera (Eds.), *Liberation psychology: Theory, method, practice, and social justice* (pp. 17–40). American Psychological Association.

Chavez, T. A., Fernandez, I. T., Hipolito-Delgado, C. P., & Rivera, E. T. (2016). Unifying liberation psychology and humanistic values to promote social justice in counseling. *The Journal of Humanistic Counseling, 55,* 166–182.

Comas-Díaz, L., & Torres Rivera, E. (Eds.). (2020). *Liberation psychology: Theory, method, practice, and social justice*. American Psychological Association.

Crenshaw, K. (1989). Demarginalizing the intersection of race and sex: A black feminist critique of antidiscrimination doctrine, feminist theory and antiracist politics. *University of Chicago Legal Forum, 140,* 139–167.

Crenshaw, K. (1991). Mapping the margins: Intersectionality, identity politics, and violence against women of color. *Stanford Law Review, 43*(6), 1241–1299.

Dekker, L. (2016). Cultural safety and critical race theory: Education frameworks to promote reflective nursing practice. In H. Brown, R. D. Sawyer & J. Norris (Eds.), *Forms of practitioner reflexivity: Critical, conversational, and arts-based approaches* (pp. 91–115). Palgrave MacMillan.

Delgado, D., & Stefancic, J. (2017). *Critical race theory: An introduction* (3rd ed.). NYU Press.

Freire, P. (1970). *Pedagogy of the oppressed*. Continuum International.

Gay, G. (2002). Preparing culturally responsive teaching. *Journal of Teacher Education, 53*, 106–116.

Gay, G. (2010). *Culturally responsive teaching: Theory, research and practice* (2nd ed.). Teachers College Press.

Gay, G. (2013). Teaching to and through cultural diversity. *Curriculum Inquiry, 43*(1), 48–70.

Gay, G. (2018). *Culturally responsive teaching: Theory, research and practice* (3rd ed.). Teachers College Press.

Goodman, L. A., Liang, B., Helms, J. E., Latta, R. E., Sparks, E., & Weintraub, S. R. (2004). Training counseling psychologists as social justice agents: Feminist and multicultural principles in action. *The Counseling Psychologist, 32*, 793–837.

Harro, B. (2000). The cycle of liberation. In M. Adams, W. Blumenfeld, R. Castaneda, H. Hackman, M. Peters & X. Zuniga (Eds.), *Readings for diversity and social justice* (pp. 618–625). Routledge.

Harro, B. (2013). The cycle of liberation. In M. Adams, W. Blumenfeld, R. Castaneda, H. Hackman, M. Peters & X. Zuniga (Eds.), *Readings for diversity and social justice* (3rd ed., pp. 463–469). Routledge.

hooks, b. (1993). A revolution of values. The promise of multi-cultural change. *Journal of the Midwest Modern Languages Association, 26*(1), 4–11.

hooks, b. (2000). *Feminist theory: From margin to center*. South End Press.

Martín-Baró, I. (1996). *Writings for a liberation psychology*. Harvard University Press.

Maté, G. (2004). *When the body says no: The cost of hidden stress*. Vintage Canada.

Ratts, M. J., Singh, A. A., Nassar-McMillan, S., Butler, S. K., & McCullough, J. R. (2015). *Multicultural and social justice counseling competencies*. Retrieved July 5, 2022, from www.counseling. org/docs/default-source/competencies/multicultural-and-social-justice-counseling-competencies.pdf?sfvrsn=20

Reyes, V., Clancy, S., Koge, H., Richardson, K., & Taylor, P. (2021). Decolonising globalised curriculum landscapes: The identity and agency of academics. *London Review of Education, 19*(1), 1–13.

Rogers, C. R. (1961). *On becoming a person*. Houghton Mifflin Company.

Samuels, A. J. (2018). Exploring culturally responsive pedagogy: Teachers' perspectives on fostering equitable and inclusive classrooms. *SRATE Journal, 21*(1), 22–30.

Singh, A. A., Appling, B., & Trepal, H. (2020). Using the multicultural and social justice counseling competencies to decolonize counseling practice: The important roles of theory, power, and action. *Journal of Counseling and Development, 98*, 261–271.

Sodhi, P. K. (2017). *Exploring immigrant and sexual minority mental health: Reconsidering multiculturalism*. Routledge.

Sodhi, P. K. (2019). Working with and supporting multicultural learners. Workshop presented at the *Kaleidoscope conference*, Algonquin College, Ottawa, Ontario, May 14–15, 2019.

Tyler, J. (2021). Decolonizing counseling practice [Audio Podcast]. *The Thoughtful Counselor*. https://concept.paloaltou.edu/?p=201727&preview=true

Index